gel-like state of the cell, created by water's structure, serves as the basis of cellular organization and function, but also that any compromise of that gel-like state can trigger the development of cancer. He connects well with readers, weaving threads of sensitivity and humanity through the fabric of the book. At the same time, he is not shy to criticize the cancer establishment for its narrow focus on genetics—which has arguably produced few gains over many decades. Highly recommended, not only for those interested in cancer—who isn't?—but also for anyone interested in logical thinking in science."

—GERALD H. POLLACK, PhD, professor,
University of Washington; author of *The Fourth Phase of Water*

"As a doctor who wholeheartedly supports a terrain-centric approach to the prevention and treatment of cancer, I found Dr. Cowan's book refreshing and inspiring. With nearly half the US population expected to have a cancer diagnosis in their lifetime, it is crucial to understand *why* in order to change these statistics. Dr. Cowan has never shied away from questioning conventional wisdom about the health-disease continuum, and this book is no different. In examining why the standard of care often falls far short of a positive outcome for those with cancer, Dr. Cowan dives into the disease's actual metabolic and cytoplasmic origins—as opposed to perceived genetic origins—and explains cancer as the result of the fundamental breakdown of a crucial element within our cells: water. For decades, many of us have been exploring a terrain-centric approach to this devastating disease process—one of damaged mitochondria, murky cytoplasm, and a deviation from our true nature. Now, with *Cancer and the New Biology of Water*, Dr. Cowan makes another important contribution to that growing body of work, bringing vitalism back into modern medicine, examining the role of structured water in cellular health, and inviting us all to consider some truly out of the box thinking to address this growing epidemic."

—DR. NASHA WINTERS, coauthor of
The Metabolic Approach to Cancer

"Dr. Cowan has written a must-read for anyone on their cancer journey. *Cancer and the New Biology of Water* is filled with research on promising treatment options that help to bridge the gap between conventional and integrative medicine."

—IVELISSE PAGE, executive director
and cofounder, Believe Big

CANCER

and the New Biology of

WATER

Also by Thomas Cowan, MD

Human Heart, Cosmic Heart:
A Doctor's Quest to Understand, Treat, and Prevent
Cardiovascular Disease

Vaccines, Autoimmunity, and the
Changing Nature of Childhood Illness

CANCER

and the New Biology of

WATER

THOMAS COWAN, MD

Foreword by Zach Bush, MD

Chelsea Green Publishing
White River Junction, Vermont
London, UK

Developmental Editor: Brianne Goodspeed
Copy Editor: Deborah Heimann
Proofreader: Nanette Bendyna
Indexer: Johanna Egert
Designer: Melissa Jacobson
Page Composition: Abrah Griggs

Printed in the United States of America.
First printing September 2019.
10 9 8 7 6 5 4 3   20 21 22 23

Our Commitment to Green Publishing
Chelsea Green sees publishing as a tool for cultural change and ecological stewardship.
We strive to align our book manufacturing practices with our editorial mission and to
reduce the impact of our business enterprise in the environment. We print our books
and catalogs on chlorine-free recycled paper, using vegetable-based inks whenever possible. This book may cost slightly more because it was printed on paper that contains
recycled fiber, and we hope you'll agree that it's worth it. *Cancer and the New Biology of
Water* was printed on paper supplied by Sheridan that contains 100% postconsumer
recycled fiber.

Library of Congress Cataloging-in-Publication Data
Names: Cowan, Thomas, 1956- author.
Title: Cancer and the new biology of water / Thomas Cowan.
Description: White River Junction, VT : Chelsea Green Publishing Company,
 [2019]
Identifiers: LCCN 2019020274 | ISBN 9781603588812 (hardcover)
 | ISBN 9781603588829 (ebook)
Subjects: LCSH: Cancer—Philosophy. | Cancer—Treatment.
Classification: LCC RC262 .C69 2019 | DDC 616.99/4—dc23
LC record available at https://lccn.loc.gov/2019020274

Chelsea Green Publishing
85 North Main Street, Suite 120
White River Junction, VT 05001
(802) 295-6300
www.chelseagreen.com

MIX
Paper from
responsible sources
FSC® C008955

The man in the street does not notice the devil
even when the devil is holding him by the throat.

—JOHANN WOLFGANG VON GOETHE

CONTENTS

Disclaimer

Cancer is a serious disease that needs to be diagnosed and treated in conjunction with your primary physician and oncologist. Nothing in this book is meant to be diagnostic or to suggest a treatment for any person with cancer. Due to current California state laws, I do not consult with or treat patients with cancer at this time. The goal of this book is to stimulate interest in a new approach to understanding cancer and cancer treatment. My hope is that as a result of this book, there will be further research into new avenues for the prevention and treatment of cancer. I also hope that individuals who seek treatment for cancer will bring up the ideas in the book to their treating physicians. But, again, nothing in this book is meant to be a prescription for treatment for any person with cancer.

FOREWORD

Mankind is now three decades into the most extraordinary chronic disease epidemic in recorded history. This global epidemic is unique for its penetration into nearly every region, culture, and socioeconomic landscape, but it is the wealthiest nations in the world that have the highest rates of chronic disease. The United States now spends about double what other high-income countries spend on health care, and yet there is no evidence that our multi-trillion-dollar annual spending has had any measurable impact on health outcomes.[1]

Despite overwhelming evidence that the pharmaceutical model is failing to reduce the chronic disease and attendant suffering that have defined recent decades, medical universities and the governmental and private entities that support them have been remarkably slow to shift thinking or allocate research budgets. The medical establishment has been resistant to exploring exciting new paradigms in our understanding of the biology of health—rather than our current industry of disease. It has therefore failed to develop treatments that would support the body's intrinsic healing capacity, and remains stuck in the "Band-Aid" approach to chronic disease management. As a result, patients unfortunately remain stuck there as well. Disease-care-as-usual doggedly marches along in a multi-trillion-dollar "health care" economy, leaving patients behind.

All the while, academic subspecialization leads to compartmentalization of knowledge among those whose charge is ostensibly to draw connections and put the medical pieces together. One of the most obvious shortcomings is the lack of cross-pollination between biology and physics in medical education. Physicians are not known for their math skills; indeed, many of us are relieved to move past the calculus and physics courses that threaten our competitive undergraduate GPAs. We cling to the concreteness of biology and pharmaceutical biochemistry, and few physicians or medical scientists have reason to return to physics in their readings, research, or clinical practice. The dilemma, of course, is that all matter in the universe—from the stars to your kitchen table and, of course, your physical body—is, at the fabric level, atomic structure, not cellular structure.

The early twentieth century was an era of scientific enlightenment with many intellectual giants and achievements in the field of physics, beyond the celebrated work of Albert Einstein. In *Cancer and the New Biology of Water*, Dr. Cowan introduces us to some of these intellectual giants, explores the relevance of their work in the context of health and the current epidemic of chronic disease, and shares therapeutic options that are now emerging from this body of work. Some of the science he covers is obscure and underappreciated, and some of it has been generated by some of the largest governmental and academic programs in history. Unfortunately, the medical community has remained seemingly unaware of, or uninterested in, the implications of these breakthroughs. When it comes to cancer therapies, chemotherapy, radiation, and surgery continue to dominate the standard of care, as well as the intellectual mind-set of most allopathic doctors and scientists. Fortunately, nature has its ways of revealing truth regardless of the attention or intention we pay to it, and nature has been busy revealing the extraordinary, and often simple, scientific truths and clinical tools that are emerging from this body of research. Today, thousands of independent scientists, physicians, intuitives, and practitioners of ancient and modern healing arts are exploring countless unconventional angles of biology and biophysics in order to better support the patients who don't have time to wait for the allopathic medical establishment to catch up.

Most of us are now only a degree of separation from a family member or close friend suffering a premature downward spiral of health. We often watch in amazement, horror, and hopelessness as health seeps out of the body while doctors, with all of our education, diagnostic tools, drug technologies, and treatments, seem unable to bring forth any meaningful therapeutic course of action, let alone a root-cause rationale for the emergence of these devastating epidemics. Too many of us are bouncing from specialist to specialist looking for answers with increasingly desperate frustration, never getting a big picture of how we came to the disorder and dysfunction of, or any meaningful solutions to, our condition.

Dr. Cowan and I share a great sense of urgency to get new perspectives on cancer into your hands because the challenges and opportunities in your life do not stop with you. Each subsequent generation since the 1960s is showing a growing burden of cancer and chronic disease, with onset happening at a younger and younger age. Time is of the essence. The efforts you make toward reversing your condition and embracing your healing potential are not just a win for your life and welfare, they can be an epicenter of change and education for your entire family and community. As such, it is my sincere hope that the following chapters will empower you to take the necessary steps to change the life you live today, and the future that you can create for yourself and those you love.

Godspeed in health and healing,

ZACH BUSH, MD
Internal Medicine, Endocrinology and
Metabolism, Hospice and Palliative Care

Introduction

In the early 1990s, a German biostatistician named Ulrich Abel published a paper that rocked the world of oncology. Abel wanted to understand what progress had been made in the twenty years since President Nixon "declared" war on cancer in 1971 with the signing of the National Cancer Act, the allocation of $1.6 billion in research funding over the next three years, and the promise of a cure within five. Nixon's optimism hadn't come out of nowhere. Researchers were trumpeting the discovery of oncogenes as the cause of cancer. It seemed as though victory was right around the corner.

Twenty years later, the United States and its global partners had poured many billions of dollars more into cancer research, and Dr. Abel wanted to understand the return on this unprecedented investment. He reviewed thousands of oncology papers published in the previous two decades and requested analysis and comments from hundreds of oncologists in order to understand the impact, specifically, of chemotherapy in the treatment of advanced epithelial cancer.[1] (Epithelial cancer makes up the majority of all cancer.) In other words, how effective is our number 1 weapon twenty years into the War on Cancer?

Dr. Abel's major finding, meticulously arrived at, was that other than lung cancer, and small-cell lung cancer in particular, there is no direct evidence that chemotherapy prolongs survival in patients with advanced carcinoma.[2] Abel went on to say that even with lung cancer, the benefit of chemotherapy is "at best rather small."[3] As Abel later stated, "Success of most chemotherapies is appalling. . . . There is no scientific evidence for its ability to extend in any appreciable way the lives of patients suffering from the most common organic cancer. . . . Chemotherapy for malignancies too advanced for surgery, which accounts for 80% of all cancers, is a scientific wasteland."[4]

To be sure, these findings raised plenty of questions. For starters, if chemotherapy confers no real benefit to patients with advanced cancer, what about those with early-stage cancer? But the findings were earth-shattering nevertheless. They directly challenged the narratives that chemotherapy is an effective weapon and that science is winning the war on cancer. According to decades of cutting-edge research, science is winning only if you don't measure whether a person actually survives, to say nothing of the misery a person undergoing chemotherapy typically endures. Essentially, with the exception of some of the less common types of cancer, Abel's review of the literature revealed that modern cytotoxic therapy does not appreciably extend the life of the patient, nor has it been shown to improve quality of life. High doses can and do shrink tumors, but this provides a questionable benefit to the patient.

As would be expected, the oncology powers that be fought against Abel's conclusions, and even attacked his character. But in doing so, they made something important very clear: Researchers often measure the success of chemotherapy by whether or not a tumor shrinks and, if so, by how much—not whether or not it prolongs the survival of the patient. The problem is that shrinkage of the tumor doesn't necessarily relate to improvement in outcomes. For example, it is well known that using anti-androgen therapy for prostate cancer (i.e., hormones) quickly selects for cancer cells that are independent of testosterone (i.e., they don't need testosterone to grow). So by giving anti-testosterone drugs, initially the tumor shrinks, and a study may measure that initial shrinkage, but the residual tumor cells "learn" to grow without testosterone, and they quickly resume growing more aggressively than the initial cancer. We see this initial shrinkage with chemotherapy treatment for other types of cancer, too.

Not everyone in the oncology community was convinced by the efforts to discredit Abel's work, however. The debate raged on for more than a decade. Then, in 2004, an independently funded literature review of randomized clinical trials evaluated the effectiveness of chemotherapy in the five-year survival rate for twenty-two major malignancies among Australian and American patients. The results? "The overall contribution of curative and adjuvant cytotoxic chemotherapy to 5-year survival in adults was estimated to be 2.3% in Australia and 2.1% in the USA." In other words, almost nothing. At the cost of an often dramatically decreased quality of life. The authors concluded that "cytotoxic chemotherapy only makes a minor contribution to cancer survival. To justify the continued funding and availability of drugs used in cytotoxic chemotherapy, a rigorous evaluation of the cost-effectiveness and impact on quality of life is urgently required." It is significant to note that the 2.3 percent and the 2.1 percent refer to all stages, not just advanced-stage cancer.[5]

By 2009, according to *New York Times* health writer Gina Kolata, the National Cancer Institute alone, to say nothing of other government agencies, universities, drug companies, and philanthropies, had spent $105 billion since the War on Cancer began, and the return on that investment was a drop in the death rate of only 5 percent between 1950 and 2005. Compare this, Kolata suggested, to the death rate for heart disease, which fell 64 percent during the same time period, or the death rate for flu and pneumonia, which fell 58 percent during the same time period. Kolata reported that only 20 percent of patients with metastatic breast cancer, 10 percent with metastatic colorectal cancer, 30 percent with metastatic prostate cancer, and fewer than 10 percent with lung cancer live more than five years. More significantly, none of these numbers has changed much in the past forty years. "Still," Kolata wrote, "the perception fed by the medical profession and its marketers, and by popular sentiment, is that cancer can almost always be prevented. If that fails, it can usually be treated, even beaten."

Not only have we failed to treat it and beat it, we seem increasingly unable to prevent it. Writing for *Newsweek* in 2018, Sylvie Beljanski noted that about one in twenty people received a cancer diagnosis at the turn of the twentieth century. By the 1940s, it was one in sixteen. By the 1970s, it was one in ten. Today, one in three people will get cancer during the course of his or her life.[6]

These numbers can be, and are, parsed ad infinitum by those who want to argue that we are winning the War on Cancer. There's a lot of incentive for championing that argument, after all. Billions of dollars of research funding, pharmaceutical drugs, and biotechnology, not to mention people's careers and reputations, and the reputations of powerful public and private institutions, are tied up in the narrative that a cure is just around the corner if we stay the course. When we think about the $4.8 billion that the American Cancer Society has invested into research since 1946 and how it trumpets a decline in mortality between 2002 and 2003, and then a decline in mortality for the second consecutive year between 2003 and 2004, it sounds promising and hopeful.[7] We want to believe it. Until we realize that the decline in mortality between 2002 and 2003 amounts to 369 people.[8] Even the larger 3,014 drop between 2003 and 2004 needs to be put into context. For the individuals who survived, it's huge. But given the 553,888 who didn't survive in 2004, or the 556,902 who didn't survive in 2003, can anyone honestly argue that the tide has turned?[9]

In 2004, cancer survivor Clifton Leaf penned a cover story for *Fortune* titled "Why We're Losing the War on Cancer (And How to Win It)" in which he explained that even the modest gain in the war has to do with public health lifestyle changes, particularly increased awareness about smoking. "Very little of this modest gain is the result of exciting new compounds discovered by the NCI labs or the big cancer research centers—where nearly all the public's money goes."

Leaf described interviewing researchers, physicians, epidemiologists, pharmacologists, biologists, and geneticists at drug companies and major research centers around the country, as well as officials at the Food and Drug Administration (FDA), National Cancer Institute (NCI), and National Institutes of Health (NIH), who collectively become for him a picture of "a dysfunctional 'cancer culture'—a groupthink that pushes tens of thousands of physicians and scientists toward the goal of finding the tiniest improvements in treatment rather than genuine breakthroughs; that fosters isolated (and redundant) problem solving instead of cooperation; and rewards academic achievement and publication over all else. At each step along the way from basic science to patient bedside, investigators rely on models that are consistently lousy at predicting success—to the point where hundreds of cancer drugs are thrust into the pipeline, and many are approved by the FDA, even though their proven 'activity' has little to do with curing cancer."[10]

I appreciate Leaf's remarks, but I would go further. I think our failure to win the War on Cancer goes way beyond "publish or perish," a dysfunctional cancer culture, the influence of Big Pharma, or the fact that thousands of people have staked their livelihood to the current model, though I think all those things are certainly factors. I think it goes way beyond the argument that cancer is a wicked problem, a wily foe whose defeat is a long, slow, tedious project (but that the wonders of science and our current methodologies will soon prevail). I think the reason we'll never win the War on Cancer on our current path is that the current path represents a fundamental misunderstanding of the nature of life, and therefore the nature of cancer. We've built an industry worth billions of dollars on this fundamental misunderstanding. The failure to cure cancer and the failure to save lives are simply its logical conclusion.

———————

There is an old joke in which a police officer comes upon a man anxiously looking for something of obvious importance under a streetlight. He asks the man what he's searching for, to which the man hurriedly answers, "My keys," and continues his desperate attempt to find them. The officer helps him look for a few minutes then stops to ask, "Where do you think you lost them?" The man replies, "In the bushes over there," nodding to the hedge a few feet away. The officer asks, "Then why are you looking over here?" The man replies, "Because the light is better here."

This book is an attempt to look in the right place for the keys to cancer. I know many mainstream scientists, researchers, and doctors vigorously dismiss those of us who stray from where the light is better, but with so many lives on the line and with such a colossal failure in plain sight, is it any wonder that the public is increasingly turning to alternative ideas and approaches? Is it not worth considering that we might be looking in the wrong place? If it is worth considering—and I believe strongly, of course, that it is—we have to go back not only to the research that was under way when Nixon announced this war, but to our very understanding of what cancer—and life—is.

PART I

A New Understanding of Cancer

CHAPTER ONE

The Failure of
the Oncogene Theory

When Nixon signed the National Cancer Act, the big news in the oncology community was the discovery of oncogenes, genes that have the capacity to cause cancer. This was followed a few years later by the discovery of proto-oncogenes, normal genes that could mutate to become oncogenes and get passed on during cell division. Sometimes these mutations are harmless, or can be repaired by the body's DNA repair processes, but sometimes they are carcinogenic and not repairable. These carcinogenic mutations lead to accelerated, uncontrolled growth, eventually leading to a proliferation of defective cells into what we call a tumor (from the Latin "to swell"). With continued growth of the defective cells we end up with disseminated or metastatic cancer and the eventual demise of the patient. The usual onco-logical strategies are directed at removing (surgery), burning out (radiation), or poisoning (chemotherapy) these fast-growing cells, with the goal of removing the cancerous growth from the body of the patient.

In medicine, we hope and expect that the therapies we use are derived directly from our understanding of the biology of the disease in treatment, so it is important to briefly describe the underlying basis of the oncogene theory, which will then allow us to understand the underpinnings of the current oncology treatments. The modern conception of the cell, built up by hundreds of years of research, is of a fatty membrane encasing a fluid-filled interior. The fluid, otherwise known as cytoplasm, is where various organelles, proteins, and other intracellular contents reside.

In the cytoplasm, these organelles carry out the orders supplied to them by the signals from the nucleus. Some organelles are involved with protein synthesis, others are involved with energy generation, still others are involved with electrolyte or fluid balance. Essentially the cytoplasm can be likened to a factory, the place where things are made under orders from management, which resides in the nucleus.

The nucleus houses the control room, DNA, which manages the cell and is the "mastermind" of all cellular processes. As most of us learned in high school, DNA is a double-helix-shaped string of nucleic acids divided into segments or genes, each of which codes the blueprint for the synthesis of its copy. Through the process of transcription, DNA provides a kind of mirror image of itself that is known as messenger RNA (mRNA). The mRNA is then transferred to the cytoplasm before the ribosomes, or protein factories, translate it into a specific protein. Proteins are the action molecules of the cell that carry out most, if not all, cellular functions. The DNA's sequence of base pairs of genes determines the protein the cell will produce. The central dogma of genetics is that each gene codes for a specific protein and the direction is always from DNA to RNA to protein, never the reverse.

There are many thousands of these genes. In a healthy state, the genes produce healthy proteins that contribute to the functionality of various processes. If, for example, a gene is coding for a protein in the retina that is involved with color vision, the result will be color vision, as long as the process produces an intact functional protein. Of course, there may be many proteins involved with color vision, in which case intact functional proteins must be produced in their optimal ratios to one another. When it comes to cell growth and division, there are thousands of genes and proteins involved in this complex process. Some of the proteins are receptors on the outside of the cell and may ferry nutrients inside or create a signal for the cell to divide. Other proteins participate in creating the spindle that pulls the chromosomes apart, allowing two new copies of the cell to form. Yet other proteins participate in other aspects of cell division.

A simple conception of the cancer process is that the cell enters the cellular growth phase too often and too readily. It has lost connection to the various feedback mechanisms that normally limit the rate and amount of cell division. The result is a disease characterized by an increase in cell division to the point where a visible tumor or new growth forms. The promise of the oncogene theory was that if we knew what a normal gene should look like on a somatic chromosome (the non-X and non-Y chromosomes) and we saw a mutation, that mutation might be responsible for inducing this proliferative change. One original hope for this theory was that we could find mutations in key genes that played critical roles in controlling the growth process. Another hope was that cancer involved the mutation in a single gene, leading to a single defective protein, that by itself drove the cancer process forward.

As research progressed from the early 1970s, researchers found many such characteristic oncogenes in all types of tumors, and when these genes were thought to be an integral part of the cell division control, it was thought (and often announced) that the gene causing a particular type of cancer had been found and that it was only a matter of time before we could figure out how to correct the gene, remove it entirely, or give the patient the "correct" protein to circumvent this faulty, cancerous process. As time went on, however, a far more complicated picture emerged in which a cancer results not from a single oncogene mutation but instead from the cumulative effects of many gene mutations affecting multiple regulatory pathways for cell division and other cellular functions.

In some cases, researchers discovered that tumors had thousands of different mutations in a single cell, many of which had some role to play in cell division. When various cells from a single individual's tumor were examined, researchers found not the clone of millions of cells each with the same single mutated gene, but a heterogeneous mixture of cells, each with their own set of mutated genes. A 2013 oncology paper gave a small glimpse into the complexity: "Malignant melanoma is the most aggressive cancer in humans and understanding this unique biological behavior may help to design better prognosticators and more efficient therapies. However, malignant melanoma is a heterogeneous tumor etiologically . . . morphologically and genetically driven by various oncogenes . . . and suppressor genes."[1]

In other words, the goal was to find the oncogenes responsible for the melanoma and indeed a number of different oncogenes affecting the growth process of melanoma have been discovered. But some of these oncogenes stimulate growth, others suppress growth, individuals with melanoma may have different oncogenes, and, even in the same individual, different cells in the tumor have different oncogenes. This situation of genetically diverse cells in one person and genetically diverse cells in one type of cancer is the rule and not the exception. In fact, there are few examples in which each cell of the cancer is genetically identical and in which individuals with the same type of cancer have cells with the same genetic makeup. The bottom line is that by looking for somatic mutations in cancer cells, we have been able to demonstrate that cancer cells are unfathomably genetically diverse among individuals with the same kind of cancer, and even within an individual's own body or tumor. Needless to say, this has made cancer therapy far more complex than what we envisioned fifty years ago.

The Failure of the Oncogene Theory

Fifty years ago the oncology community bet the farm on the idea that the root cause of cancer was to be found in genetic mutations and that if we could find the mutated genes in an individual's cancer cells or if we could find a specific mutation associated with a certain type of cancer, we would be well on our way to a cure. This is where the light was shining brightest, so this is where we looked. And we were committed to a concept of biology in which DNA controls our cellular function, and therefore our health.

The story of this book is that both of these theories are tragically flawed. The somatic mutations seen in cancer cells are the result of a cellular deterioration that has little to do with oncogenes, DNA, or even the nucleus of a cell. Furthermore, the concept of DNA as masterminding the life of the cell, controlling its every move, is wrong. Rather, DNA is one aspect of the complex life of the cell and the life of the organism. It is essential to rethink science's obsessive focus on DNA and genetic determinism if we are ever to make real strides in the prevention and treatment of this devastating disease.

How is it even possible that our federal government, academic institutions, and gigantic research corporations could have poured billions of dollars into pursuing a faulty theory of this disease? I know it seems improbable. Impossible. But try to suspend your disbelief long enough to recall the results we are seeing after fifty years of intense research and chemotherapy's dismal statistics. And then add this to it: For the majority of common cancers—breast, prostate, pancreas—the fifty-year search for oncogenes has not changed the treatment of these cancers. Rather than living in an age of bio-individual, oncogene-based treatment, we are still using the same old triad: removing (surgery), burning out (radiation), or poisoning (chemotherapy). In almost no cases is cancer treated in a manner inspired by our search for oncogenes. In other words, in large measure the oncogene has borne almost no fruit with regard to treatment. It is reasonable—indeed, necessary—to ask ourselves whether we are on the right track.

Granted, there are many new cancer treatments that have been brought to market, especially in the past decade. Most are "targeted therapies," targeting one or more of the oncogenes we are discussing. We are supposedly on the cusp of a breakthrough in the treatment of cancer as a result of these new, targeted therapies. But what do studies of these breakthrough therapies actually reveal?

A 2017 paper published in *JAMA Oncology* presented some stunning conclusions. Of sixty-two new oncology drugs approved between 2003 and 2013, only 43 percent offered a survival benefit of three months or longer, 11 percent offered a survival benefit of less than three months, 15 percent had an unknown survival benefit, and 30 percent offered no survival benefit at all.[2] Furthermore, 45 percent were associated with reduced patient safety.[3]

A 2017 study published in the *British Medical Journal* (*BMJ*) that looked at the survival and quality-of-life benefits of forty-eight cancer drugs approved in Europe by the European Medicines Agency (EMA) between 2009 and 2013 reached similar conclusions: "This systematic evaluation of oncology approvals by the EMA in 2009–13 shows that most drugs entered the market without evidence of benefit on survival or quality of life. At a minimum of 3.3 years after market entry, there was still no conclusive evidence that these drugs either extended or improved life for most cancer indications. When there were survival gains over existing treatment options or placebo, they were often marginal."[4]

While the *JAMA Oncology* paper and the *BMJ* paper looked at survival and quality of life, it's important to understand that many studies done on new drugs that reportedly target oncogenes don't evaluate their efficacy in the context of survival or quality of life. For example, the *BMJ* review noted that only 26 percent of the studies were using survival as their primary end point.[5]

The rest used surrogate markers. Surrogate markers mean that if a patient has, for example, a 5 × 5 centimeter tumor in the pancreas and a treatment shrinks that tumor to 1×1 centimeters, the treatment can be considered effective based on its effect on the tumor. The problem is that the oncology literature is full of documentation that successfully shrinking a tumor doesn't necessarily translate to a better outcome for the patient. The toxicity to the patient based on the use of the drug might mean that the patient actually dies sooner and experiences a worse quality of life than if no treatment at all had been given.

In other words, surrogate markers can be a worse-than-useless way of evaluating a new cancer therapy because the results can be framed to make the therapy look effective even if it kills the patient. And yet, in the studies that the *BMJ* paper reviews, only one-quarter of the new "targeted" cancer therapies studied overall survival or quality of life. In 69 percent of the cases, approval of the new drugs was based on studies done on surrogate markers, meaning that they provided no real information on whether the drugs actually worked in terms of improving outcomes for the *patients*. Consider this carefully the next time you hear about the promise of new, "targeted" cancer drugs.[6]

Finally, we need to address the message that while we still have a long road ahead in identifying the oncogenes at play in certain common cancers, some oncogenes have been identified, they are medical breakthroughs, and the discoveries should give everyone confidence that science is on the right track. The most famous example is *BRCA*, the breast cancer gene, which prompted Angelina Jolie (and thousands of other women) to undergo a double mastectomy. People who carry it, we hear, are at high risk of developing aggressive breast cancer. It is proof, we hear, that a single gene mutation can cause cancer, and we can therefore believe that given time, and further investment, we'll find a similar gene for all the other kinds of cancer.

The rub is that this conclusion isn't shared by everyone who's researching this topic in depth. A 2018 paper published in *The Lancet Oncology* looked at women forty years old and younger who developed young-onset breast cancer to determine the effect of a *BRCA1* or *BRCA2* mutation on outcomes. The study's authors concluded that "[There is] no significant difference in overall survival or distant disease-free survival between patients carrying a *BRCA1* or *BRCA2* mutation and patients without these mutations after a diagnosis of breast cancer."[7] The authors go on to state, "We found no clear evidence that either *BRCA1* or *BRCA2* germline mutations significantly affect overall survival with breast cancer after adjusting for known prognostic factors."[8] Unlike the death sentence we are told is conferred by the *BRCA* mutation, in fact, the *BRCA* mutation is heterogeneous and some of its variations may actually be protective. As the authors of a 2011 paper titled "The Case against BRCA 1 and 2 Testing," published in the journal *Surgery*, stated, "A variation in K1183R is related *inversely* to cancer risk. It seems that some polymorphisms may actually have a protective effect."[9]

A 2015 meta-analysis of sixty-six studies on the *BRCA* gene mutation concluded that "in contrast to currently held beliefs of many oncologists and despite 66 published studies, it is not yet possible to draw evidence-based conclusions about the association between *BRCA1* and/or *BRCA2* mutation carriership and breast cancer prognosis."[10] In other words, the preponderance of the evidence concerning the *BRCA* gene mutations is that they have very little effect on the prognosis for those carrying this mutation. I had to wonder during the media storm of Jolie's decision whether the press coverage and public "education" about *BRCA1* and *BRCA2* that surrounded it were in fact a calculated public relations campaign for a failing therapy as opposed to real information that could help real people and prevent real suffering.

Finally, we turn our attention to the "star" of the oncogenetic world, the drug Gleevec, a targeted therapy for a rare form of leukemia called chronic myelogenous leukemia (CML), which is considered the purest example of a single mutation creating a distinct kind of cancer. Gleevec interferes with the expression of this gene and quickly and dramatically causes remission with no damage to the normal cells. This result was, and is, hailed as the strongest possible proof of the oncogene theory. You can appreciate the enthusiasm, tempered with a bit of caution, concerning the discovery of Gleevec:

> *In a way, Gleevec is an exceptional case, and the same success is not likely to be achieved with other cancers any time soon. Unlike most other cancers, which are caused by a multitude of complex interacting genetic and environmental factors and therefore have many targets, CML is caused by a single aberrant protein related to a consistent chromosomal translocation. Scientists were thus able to focus all of their efforts on this single target. Nonetheless, the Gleevec story is no less an excellent and, some would say, beautiful example of how knowledge of the biological functioning of a cell can lead to life-saving medical treatment.* [11]

It is important to give credit where credit is due and to applaud a breakthrough in cancer treatment, even if it is for a rare form of the disease. The interesting footnote of the Gleevec story, however, is that in the past few years reports have emerged that there are two other commonly used medical drugs that also have a dramatically curative effect on patients with CML, and neither affects the oncogene that is supposedly responsible for the disease. Rather, both drugs share a molecular three-dimensional shape with the Gleevec molecule that has left researchers wondering if this is the actual reason that Gleevec is effective against CML. In other words, even the miracle of Gleevec for CML may have another, simpler, more accurate explanation than its effect on an oncogene.

This curious possibility that it is the "shape" of Gleevec that confers its effectiveness is a potent reminder that there are other possible explanations for cancer. The biggest "other possible explanation" of all is that maybe the oncogene theory—which is the foundation of the biotech industry—is wrong. Or, more fairly stated, maybe the oncogene therapy is, at best, a superficial understanding of the biology of cancer. What if cancer is not primarily a genetic disease? What if the hundreds, even thousands, of somatic mutations that have by now been found associated with cancer cells are not the *cause* of cancer but are a *symptom* of underlying processes that have led to the degeneration of the cellular environment? If that's the case, what events lead a healthy cell to become a cancer cell—and what is the "location" of those events? Is there an identifiable mechanism that can lead from cellular abnormalities to an increase in somatic mutations?

CHAPTER TWO

The Locus of Cancer

The question of whether we have misplaced the "location" of cancer in the nucleus of a cell is actually surprisingly easy to answer from a scientific standpoint, having been worked out in large part for about a century, first with the work of Dr. Otto Warburg and more recently with the work of Dr. Thomas Seyfried. The most important organelle to understand when it comes to the etiology of cancer is not the nucleus, but the mitochondria. The cell, like any system in nature, needs energy to do work. Work, in this case, refers to any process in the cell. Mitochondria are the energy factories of the cell that fuel these processes. Thought to originate from primitive bacteria that eons ago merged with the developing mammalian cells via symbiogenesis, these mitochondria are the site of oxidative phosphorylation, the process our cells use to produce the energy needed to run all their functions.

The goal and steps of the oxidative phosphorylation process are to generate ATP, the energy molecule used by the cell to fuel all other cellular processes. Oxidative phosphorylation generates thirty-six ATP molecules for each glucose molecule that enters the pathway. Simply put, our cells use glucose to produce energy via a biochemical pathway housed in our mitochondria, but we also have a second pathway for generating energy, glycolysis (essentially fermentation), which is crucial to understanding the genesis of cancer. This glycolytic pathway is used by primitive organisms such as yeast to generate energy, and mammalian cells will switch to the glycolytic pathway instead of oxidative phosphorylation when there is not enough oxygen and oxidative phosphorylation cannot proceed, or when there is some defect in the oxidative phosphorylation pathway itself.

The glycolytic pathway is much less efficient in generating ATP than oxidative phosphorylation. In fact, glycolysis generates only two molecules of ATP per glucose molecule, as opposed to the thirty-six generated through oxidative phosphorylation. Furthermore, glycolysis doesn't fully break down glucose into water and carbon dioxide (CO_2), as oxidative phosphorylation does; the glycolytic pathways produce toxic by-products, including alcohol and lactic acid. While this is good for wine and beer production, it is not good for our cells. This process is known as the Warburg effect, after the German doctor, physiologist, and Nobel laureate Otto Warburg, who first described it in 1924.

When I describe this to my patients—that oxidative phosphorylation occurs in the mitochondria and generates thirty-six units of ATP per molecule of glucose versus the glycolytic pathway, which occurs in the cytoplasm and generates only two—I tell them it's akin to having a job that pays $36 per hour until your boss suddenly says that, due to changes in the company, your new salary is $2 per hour. Unless you quit and look for new work, your only choice is to work eighteen times as hard to generate the same livable income. For most people, this simply wouldn't be possible. The same is true of our cells. When they find themselves relying on glycolysis to generate their energy needs, they will also find themselves in a rapidly escalating chronic shortfall. It simply isn't possible to keep up.

In most cells, approximately 40 percent of the energy they generate is used for mitosis. Another 40 percent maintains proper electrolyte balance, in particular the balance of sodium and potassium on the inside and outside of the cell. Cell division and the distribution of ions across the cell membrane are fundamental functions in the life of the cell. A cell that doesn't divide is destined to be a dead cell. A cell that cannot maintain the proper ionic gradient across its membrane loses it charge and is unable to integrate into the surrounding tissue and organ. A cell with an energy deficit is analogous to a homeowner whose mortgage is $30,000 per month and who earns a salary of $1,500 per month. Catastrophe is just around the corner.

This explains the ability of positron emission tomography (PET) scans to diagnose cancer. In a PET scan, the patient is injected with radioactive glucose. Since cancer cells are energy-starved cells and need access to about eighteen times as much glucose as a normal cell to generate the same amount of energy, they will "upregulate" every available mechanism to gain access to more glucose. Naturally, they never succeed in getting eighteen times the usual amount, but they do increase their glucose uptake enough to light up on the PET scan. The cells that take up this excessive amount of glucose are the cancer cells. We routinely use this diagnostic tool to help us detect nests of cancer cells located at various sites around the body. This should leave us with no doubt that energy generation is one of the most characteristic aspects of the cancer process.

Dr. Thomas Seyfried, cancer researcher and professor of biology at Boston College, has done the most important recent work in establishing that cancer is, first and foremost, a metabolic disease, rather than a genetic disease arising from abnormalities in the nucleus and DNA. In his seminal book *Cancer as a Metabolic Disease*, Dr. Seyfried outlines years of experimentation in which researchers transplanted nuclei from both healthy cells and cancer cells into the cytoplasm of both healthy cells and cancerous cells. What the researchers consistently found was that if you transplant the nucleus—the place where the DNA and specifically, in cancer, mutated DNA is found—from healthy cells into the cytoplasm of healthy cells, you get progeny that are healthy cells. Unsurprisingly, they also found that if you transplant the nuclei of cancerous cells, which contain the somatic mutations we are told cause cancer, into the cytoplasm of cancerous cells, you get progeny that are cancerous.

But here's where it gets interesting: When researchers transplant nuclei from cancer cells into cells with healthy cytoplasm, the resulting progeny were healthy cells with no sign of cancer. When researchers reversed direction and transplanted healthy nuclei from noncancerous cells into the cytoplasm of cancerous cells, the resulting progeny were cancerous cells.[1] Interestingly, the researchers speculate on possible mechanisms that enabled the cytoplasm to "heal" the mutations that occurred in the cancerous nuclei.

In other words, they don't seem to entertain the possibility that somatic mutations don't drive cancer to begin with. This example shows how powerful the genetic paradigm is: It determines what we are able to see and how we interpret the facts.

If we accept that these are the crucial events underlying the development of cancer, the next step is to determine if we can discover an effective approach to deprive the cancer cells of glucose, while still feeding the normal cells. This would help rebalance the energy dynamics that lie at the heart of cancer. This usually means exploring the ketogenic diet and various drugs and supplements that affect blood glucose or that interfere with the ability of the cancer cells to take up the enormous quantities of glucose they require.

The basis of these interventions is that because of cancer cells' massive need for glucose, they by necessity forgo metabolic flexibility and put all their eggs into the glycolysis basket, so to speak. Normal, healthy cells, having much less need for glucose, don't have to do this and therefore still retain the ability to use fats and proteins as sources of fuel. The ketogenic diet eliminates carbohydrates (glucose) from the diet. When the ketogenic diet is used as an intervention for cancer, the theory is that this will starve the cancer cells while allowing healthy cells to use abundantly supplied fats as fuel. Though this sounds promising and, in fact, is beginning to show signs of helping many cancer patients, there are still flaws in this theory and practice.

The main flaw, noted by Seyfried himself, is that no matter how few carbohydrates or even how little food someone eats—even if patients go on a complete water fast for days—the body's mechanisms for blood-sugar regulation keep blood glucose from dropping to levels that would be effective in killing cancer cells. This is why Dr. Seyfried seems adamant that we need to use blood-sugar-lowering drugs or medicines to augment fasting and the ketogenic diet. Unfortunately, no such safe or reliable drug exists.

I am all for pursuing the dietary and medicine approach based on exploiting the metabolic inflexibility of the cancer cells, and I believe more research should be done in this important subject, but I also think we need to further develop our understanding of the events in the cytoplasm. Now that we have located the cancer process in the cytoplasm and identified the nature of the defect arising there as one of energy needs and availability in the cell, our next step is to go deeper into the nature of the cytoplasm to see if we can also understand the nature of healing and wholeness in our patients suffering from cancer. This is where we begin to deviate even further from where the light is, and we begin to think very differently about the nature of health and disease, what we know about biology, and the nature of life.

We are erroneously taught early in life that matter can only exist in one of three "states": solid, liquid, or gaseous. For example, copper can exist as solid copper (often mixed with other elements), molten or liquid copper, or, when exposed to extreme heat, gaseous copper. There is no other state possible; the transition is from one state to the next with no intermediate steps. The transformation occurs mainly under the influence of heat, but influences such as pressure may also play a role.

If we apply this concept to water, then we can conclude that water can only exist as ice (solid), water (liquid), or steam (gas). We were all taught this in elementary school science class. The problem, like so many "truths" in science (and frankly in our culture in general), is that it doesn't stand up to even a cursory examination. In this case, we have all seen and probably eaten Jell-O, which is composed of over 90 percent water yet clearly is in none of the above three states. In fact, the state of matter that a substance assumes is not a vague concept; it can be clearly demonstrated with apparatuses that measure the bond angle between the individual molecules. Ice has a distinct bond angle between each molecule, water has a different bond angle, and in steam the molecules are mostly unattached to the other molecules. The gel that makes up Jell-O has none of these bond angles. Instead it has an intermediate bond angle that is characteristic of the gel state. Dr. Gerald Pollock, in his seminal book *The Fourth Phase of Water*, describes in detail the formation and characteristics of this fourth phase. That it exists is not in dispute. The issue is that it is not recognized for the importance that it has to the entire field of biology.

Water is the only "substance" that can exist in this fourth state, at least as far as I know. This fourth phase of water, also called structured water, is the basis of biological life.

I first started questioning the three-states-of-matter dogma when I started working as an ER doctor. We, of course, had been taught that every cell contains about 70 percent water. This was easily proven, and then no further mention was made of the water. In other words, after this cursory mention, the role and state of water were completely ignored. We just assumed it must be liquid water. But in the ER I saw hundreds of people with traumatic injuries—bullet wounds, stabbings, and other terrible wounds—but I never once saw any water squirting out of a wounded person, nor any puddle of water lying on the floor next to the injured patient. Where was the water? Blood, yes, but I had just spent years being told that humans are basically a bag of water with stuff dissolved in it, yet clearly there is no water in any cell in our bodies.

Reading the work of Dr. Pollack and of cell physiologist and biochemist Dr. Gilbert Ling years later finally cleared up this mystery. All of the "water" in our cells is in the fourth, or structured, phase. As with Jell-O, you can poke holes in it or squish it and you will never see "water" squirt out because the water is held together in a gel matrix. Jell-O is formed through the interaction of a hydrophilic surface (in this case the gelatin proteins), water, and then a heat source. The role of heat in producing Jell-O is to unfold the proteins so that they can attach to the water molecules. Without the heat the proteins remain tightly folded and can't bond to water and no gel forms. Upon cooling, the characteristic gel forms. The water inside of our cells is similar. You start with water and add protein (some evidence exists that the protein is actin, one of the main structural proteins in the body), which then together form the characteristic fourth-state gel.

What about the heat? Obviously we can't add direct heat to this system to unfold the proteins.

What Ling discovered is that ATP, the so-called energy molecule, does not produce energy at all but rather plays the role of heat in biological systems. Specifically, ATP binds to the end of the intracellular structural proteins, unfolding them, therefore allowing them to bind with the water in the cells to form gels. Without ATP, no gel forms and the function of the cell collapses. This vital but misunderstood role of ATP in biological systems will become crucial in our understanding of the cancer process.

The integrity of the intracellular gel has a role in every important function carried out by the cell. It is the foundation of life itself and the manifestation or embodiment of what I will be calling the life force of the organism. For example, when it is formed properly in a clear, crystalline, correct bond angle "structure," the intracellular mesh, because of its specific size, inherently binds to potassium inside the cell and excludes the sodium. As I explained in my 2018 book *Vaccines, Autoimmunity, and the*

Changing Nature of Childhood Illness, this is the real sodium-potassium pump—not the mostly irrelevant pump that exists in the cell membrane. Nature has been so organized that the gel itself, with no energy needed, creates and supports this important distribution of potassium inside and sodium outside the cell. As a result, the cell becomes charged, is able to "do work," and, because it then carries a charged "halo" at its exterior, is able to assume proper spatial orientation with other cells. In other words, without the healthy sodium-potassium gradient, a cell loses its charge and, like a battery, becomes a dead cell. A dead cell loses its "halo," clumps together with other cells, and forms the characteristic tumor that is one of the hallmarks of cancer.

Another function of the intracellular gels is to provide spatial orientation to the protein or DNA structures in our cells. In other words, proteins and DNA function because they assume a particular and functional three-dimensional shape inside the cell. This shaping is a direct result of the cell's interaction with water. For example, through the Human Genome Project, we learned that DNA contains about 30,000 functional genes. As the action sites of the DNA, genes are the unit that codes for the individual protein. We once thought that each gene coded for one and only one specific protein, but then we found out that there are at least 200,000 proteins in our cells. The question was, how do 30,000 genes code for 200,000 proteins? It's like a game of scrabble. A gene is like the letters *T*, *E*, and *A*. This makes the word (or protein) *tea*. But it can also make *eat* or even *ate*; it depends on the "consciousness" of the player. Now we know there are cutting and splicing proteins that actually determine the order of the letters in our genes, but the determining factor in how a gene will be expressed lies in the structured gel within which the DNA resides, not in the DNA itself. In other words, the gel structure of the water is the consciousness of the player in the Scrabble game. This means that the expression of our DNA, the very thing modern oncology is so focused on, is nothing more than a result of a properly formed and functioning gel structure in the cell.

The "reason" nature chose water to play this fundamental role in our biology is that structured water has two unique and fundamental properties. The first is that it has infinite binding sites, and the second is that when anything binds with this intracellular crystalline gel structure, it can produce instantaneous effects throughout the entire cell. The way to picture this is to imagine a window blind that can exist in either an open (lets light in) or closed (darkness) state. One simple turn of the lever or pull on the string and the entire blind changes state. The intracellular gel binds to hormones, chemicals, emotions, thoughts, and on and on; each creates subtle changes in its configuration, which is then translated into a specific action by the cell. For example, if you put estrogen in the cell, it binds with intracellular gel, subtly changing it; this then creates the unfolding of the DNA so that it facilitates the expression of the part of the DNA that codes for proteins that produce breast tissue. In this way, exposure to estrogen creates the effect desired by the cell. Humans interact with and are impacted by an infinite number of stimuli. Our ability to accept these stimuli and turn them into action is a function of our intracellular gels. This is the case whether we're talking about chemicals or deep spiritual impulses. Nothing turns into action without impacting our intracellular gels.

This understanding then allows a working definition of health and disease. Health is the state of perfect intracellular gels. Disease is when this gel state deteriorates. It is then no wonder that good food, healthy water, sunshine, interaction with the earth, love, and acceptance—all of which produce healthier, more robust intracellular gel—improve our health. In contrast, interaction with glyphosate, electromagnetic fields, and toxic chemicals deteriorates our gels and makes us sick. This book is fundamentally an exploration of how things affect our intracellular gels and, in the end, can either result in or heal us from the disease state called cancer.

My medical training was unusual, something I'm grateful for today, decades later. One of the things I learned during the course of it is that in order to become an anthroposophical physician, it is not sufficient to know biology and medicine. You must have a much broader understanding of life, and the world. My mentor, Dr. Otto Wolff, used to say that an anthroposophical doctor has to know everything. This is unattainable, of course, but I was continually amazed that Dr. Wolff seemed to know every star, every plant, every mineral, every biochemical pathway, every important painting, every significant musical composition (and could play many of them on either the violin or the piano) and spoke at least ten languages fluently, including a few ancient languages that allowed him to read esoteric works in their original language. Johann Wolfgang von Goethe, the person Rudolf Steiner considered the true founder of anthroposophy, considered one of his main achievements to be the founding of a way of seeing the world that, if followed, can lead to incredible insights. Goethe taught that his method, sometimes referred to as Goetheanistic observation, is a technique that allows one to "read" the book of nature. That is, one must let the phenomena speak for themselves with as little bias or interpretation from the observer as possible.

Modern scientists tend to study nature in the opposite way, although it espouses objectivity. If we want to know about the plant called dandelion, we start by naming the plant, stating what family of plants it belongs to, and then we describe the details of the plant we think are relevant to understanding it. We say the plant has an annual growth habit, it contains this amount of potassium, a different amount of nitrogen, and reproduces in this certain fashion. At the end of our study of the dandelion we may know a lot of details about the plant, we may even know how to grow it or get rid of it, but we don't really know the plant. It is hard to describe an essence of anything, but to practice Goetheanistic observation, you have to come to the dandelion with as few preconceptions as possible and then experience its changing nature as it progresses through time.

With the dandelion first we see a nondescript, low-growing plant that, at least for me, evokes no reaction. At this point in the life of the plant, I find nothing that interests me about this plant. Then seemingly out of nowhere, a stalk shoots up with an appealing bright yellow flower. I wouldn't say beautiful, like some other flowers, just appealing. Children, in particular, seem to have an affinity for dandelion flowers, often popping them off their thick stems in the middle of a game of tag. Then the dandelion flower disappears, almost overnight, and leaves behind a seed puffball that looks like a kind of flower skeleton, or scaffolding. I can't think of another plant flower that leaves such an intact skeletal system in its place. This skeleton flower is also attractive; I can remember spring days from my childhood spent picking and blowing them apart. I can't say why I did this, except it just seemed like the thing to do with a dandelion flower. Everyone did it.

This childhood game is Goetheanistic observation, interaction with different aspects of nature as you develop a personal relationship with and experience of your subject. Only once this more intimate connection is formed can you bring these experiences into the realm of thinking as you try to understand why the plant has "chosen" to live in this manner. At that point, you begin to understand the essence of the plant. And I would contend it is only at this point that you can understand and use the plant for healing purposes. Until then it is just "book-learning," a superficial understanding, based on how we name and categorize things, but not based on much understanding of a thing itself. In this way, most children know more about dandelions than most scientists.

This superficial understanding leads us to use plant medicines as we would use drugs. For example, instead of using aspirin to thin the blood in a person at risk of stroke, we might use a plant extract from ginkgo leaves because of the blood-thinning effect of the chemical ginkgolides. A Goetheanistically thinking physician, however, might experience the person in her office as struggling with the ravages of aging. Looking out into nature to find a healing agent for this person who is at risk of suffering from one of the many effects of aging she might look to the ginkgo tree as a being that has "learned" how to overcome, as far as this is possible, the aging process. As a physician you can "re-unite" the person suffering from premature aging with the leaves of the ginkgo tree, perhaps the longest lived plant on earth. Wholeness is achieved and the patient will hopefully experience relief.

If we apply these Goetheanistic principles to the study of cancer, coming at the problem with as few preconceptions as possible, we can observe two properties that are found in all cancer cells. The first observable property is that the tumor (in solid cancers, which are the vast majority) does not feel like the surrounding tissue. The cancer feels too dense, too hard, and quite unlike the normal, softer feel of the surrounding tissue. How does this abnormal density of the cancerous growth arise? Normally the cells that make up any of the bodily tissues assume a spatial orientation with regard to the other cells so that they maintain proper distance from each other. As a result of proper spacing, the collection of cells creates an organ with a characteristic and healthy density.

The spacing of the cells is a function of the charge generated around the cell. This charge around the cell is the result of the distribution of sodium (Na) and potassium (K) across the cell membrane. By excluding Na from the cell and accumulating K within the cell, the cell generates a halo of negative charges around itself, which creates the normal spatial orientation seen in the tissue when it contacts other similarly negatively charged cells. The separation of Na and K inside and outside the cell, while usually thought to be a function of an embedded Na+/K+ pump in the cell membrane, is in fact a result of certain properties of water.[2]

Because cancer cells are in a state of chronic energy deficiency, they are unable to properly exclude Na and accumulate K as they should, leading to a weak or absent charge around the cell. Cells with weak or absent charges clump together, leading to the characteristic density of the cancer growth. The rocklike feel is due to the increased density of the cancerous cells because they lack the usual charge around the cell and therefore are unable to assume their normal orientation. We will see later that Dr. Max Gerson developed a successful cancer therapy based on this idea of restoring the healthy charge around the cell as the key to addressing the problem of cancer. We will also see that once we develop a clearer understanding of the role of water in producing this Na+/K+ gradient, we will also get a clear picture of how to heal this defect in the cancer cell.

The second observable property of cancer cells is that, unlike normal cells, cancer cells have an abnormal number of chromosomes. The number of chromosomes found in each cell is one of the most defining aspects of a given species. Humans have forty-six chromosomes, twenty-two pairs of somatic chromosomes and one set consisting of either an XX (female) or XY (male). Fruit flies have four chromosomes, dogs have thirty-nine, and rice plants have twelve. A cancer cell is identified as such due to an abnormal number of chromosomes. This is called an aneuploid cell, as opposed to a normal or diploid cell, and the abnormality is present in all cancer cells. This simple, clear observation is verifiable by anyone with access to cancerous cells and a microscope.

What this abnormality suggests is that, if the number of chromosomes defines the species, in a way, cancer cells are not properly human cells. Healthy cells demonstrate an impulse to fit into the overall organization of the organism. Cancer cells have no such impulse. Being a species of their own, cancer cells try to create their own separate organism with no regard for the health of the whole. This is one reason cancer poses such a threat to the body.

How does this aneuploid cell form? What leads to its genesis? If we go back to the energy dynamics of the cell, we see that up to 40 percent of the energy of the cell is devoted to cell division, or mitosis. Cancer cells are energy-starved cells, which leads them to make mistakes, even huge mistakes in cell division. Sometimes the chromosomes don't separate properly; other times the spindle that "drags" half the chromosomes to one side, half to the other side, doesn't function properly; there are many other possibilities for error. Furthermore, during the process of cell division, the genes, comprising the chromosomes, are exposed to external mutagenic influences (for example, chemicals, radiation, low nutrient levels, glyphosate) leading to the high levels of mutations seen in cancer cells. The bottom line is that the energy dynamics of the cancer cell show us how cancer cells become aneuploid cells and why they have so many more somatic mutations than a healthy cell. In this light, the cancer process can begin to come into focus.

If we have cells without the proper spatial orientation, but they are diploid (have a normal number of chromosomes), we have a benign tumor or a cyst. If we generate aneuploid cells that cannot maintain proper spatial relationships to other cells, we have a malignant tumor. The clinical disease we call cancer occurs when there is a combination of these two defects, aneuploid cells that cannot support proper spatial orientation.

If it is the case that cancer is metabolically driven, rather than genetically driven, and furthermore, if it is the case that cancer results from distorted structure of the intracellular water, then we need a radically new understanding of biology in order to correctly approach it. Solving the puzzle of cancer is important not only because the disease so dramatically affects the lives of so many people and so many families. It is important also because understanding cancer can lead us to a better understanding of biology—the study of life—and that has implications for every disease, every organism, and every ecosystem. Our current model is failing because it offers no significant understanding of the simple and profound question "What is life?" Without this insight, cancer cannot be understood or properly treated. Cancer doesn't care if it is easier to study oncogenes and somatic mutations, if that is not where the true cause of the imbalance lies. If we've lost our keys in the bushes, no matter how little light or how many thorns there are in those bushes, that is where we must look.

CHAPTER THREE

What Is Life?

When I say we must begin to gain a greater understanding of the question "What is life?" it seems like a huge and an undoable task. It is my opinion, however, that we know enough to make a significant positive impact in the life of a person confronting cancer. When I have this conversation with my patients, I often start by asking them to imagine a carrot lying on the cutting board. Try to picture what this carrot is made of, I tell them. It has water, fiber, vitamins, and many other chemicals. Then go deeper: What are all those substances made of? The answer, of course, is various atoms that have arranged themselves in the form of molecules that make up the substance of the carrot. Now, imagine all of those atoms having lost their connection to each other, including the water, so what we have left is a certain number of all the various atoms that go into the making of the carrot. In other words, we have—and to be clear, this is pure conjecture to make a point—3 trillion hydrogen atoms, 1.5 million oxygen atoms, 2 trillion carbon atoms, 0.5 trillion sulfur atoms, and so on. Any chemist or, for that matter, any oncologist would tell you that the substance that constitutes a carrot is the entirety of the carrot.

Now imagine you called up the local chemical supply company and ordered this same number of atoms in the identical ratio that made up a carrot and had it delivered to your house. You open the box and pour it onto your cutting board. Is it a carrot? This heap of atoms clearly has all the substances that make up a carrot. We are told by modern science that substance is all that exists, so if all the substance is there, it should be a carrot. Does it have the same taste as a carrot, the same smell, the same nutrition? If you did the same analysis for a beet and came out with slightly different numbers and ratios for the beet as opposed to the carrot, is the sole difference between a carrot and a beet to be found in this different composition of nutrients?

My guess is that most people reading this are quite sure that the heap of atoms constituting the substance of a carrot is not the same thing as a carrot. In fact, I would venture to say that most people reading this would agree that the heap of atoms is missing the very thing that makes a carrot a carrot—a plant worthy of our care and attention, because it is distinct, knowable, and valuable to us. Lastly, I predict that most people reading this would agree that the difference between a carrot and a beet is not to be found in their differing amounts or ratios of atoms. I don't know, of course, but this is my strong suspicion.

I'm not claiming that the substance that makes up a carrot, or a human cell, is irrelevant. Whatever it is we call a carrot has an affinity to uptake more sulfur from the soil than whatever it is we call a beet. Yet, I also know that the thing that makes a carrot a carrot, a beet a beet, or any living organism that particular living organism does not lie in parsing out the chemicals it is made of. Carrots, beets, and cells, including cancer cells, are living beings, and the distinctive nature of each of these living beings is to be found somewhere beyond the physical matter of it. This other "stuff," whatever it turns out to be, is what we call life. It is where the action is, it is the key to understanding biology and the key to understanding health, disease, and cancer in particular.

Science has no good definition of life, no conception of life, and is frankly antagonistic to anyone who thinks "What is life?" should be the first and most important question. Science believes in substance, in matter, in the material world, even though we have no real clue how matter forms itself into either a carrot or a human being or an elephant or a cancer cell. Try as we might, we have not made progress in our understanding of how consciousness arises out of a collection of atoms.

Yet some things about life stand out and are very clear. The first is that in order for there to be life there must be water. No life has ever arisen, or will ever rise, out of a completely desiccated, water-free environment. In other words, when we are breaking down our carrot into its constituent atoms, the first molecule that must be broken and eliminated is water. Where there is water, there will also be life. This is significant.

The second thing that's clear about life is that the water brings a certain form to the collection of atoms. There are many differences between the carrot and the heap of atoms, but the most striking difference is that the carrot has a form, the beet has a different form, your liver has yet another form, and the form of your liver is distinct from the form of your eye. This is also significant.

The third thing that's clear about life is that this combination of water and form gives rise to unique qualities. These qualities are related to the molecules they are composed of. For example, the perfume industry rests on the knowledge that certain molecules evoke certain qualities of smell. The food industry rests on the knowledge that other molecules evoke certain qualities of taste. In the carrot, these characteristic molecules exist in the cells and tissues of the carrot. These cells and tissues are a product of this forming, or life impulse, on a molecular level. Qualities, therefore, are among the properties of whatever it is that gives rise to life. That is, the qualities of taste, smell, texture, and nutrients are part of the substance we call a carrot, which is distinct, knowable, and—in the case of carrots, and other things we choose to include in our lives—valuable.

When we leave out the nonmatter component of the study of living things, we are actually leaving out precisely what makes each distinct, knowable, and valuable in the context of other living things. Science and medicine, as currently practiced in most of the United States, and increasingly around the world, are attempting to understand health and disease while shortcutting around the most important consideration of what life is. It's an impossible task and a bizarre, unfathomable oversight. If we are ever to understand health and disease, I believe we must restore this question to its rightful place as the central concept of an effective medical system. I think it will unlock new avenues and insights in our pursuit of understanding the cause of cancer, as well as therapies that can safely and effectively address cancer. The usual explanations, even the metabolic approach, are only a part of the story. Because we only know about part of this story, the aspects that lead to healing are poorly understood. So, again, we have to start asking different questions—*very* different questions—in the practice and study of medicine.

Over the years, for example, I have had a number of medical students and young doctors shadow me in my office. Most were interested in learning about either anthroposophical medicine, in particular, or holistic medicine, more generally. Years ago, when I was living and practicing in New Hampshire, my friend's son got permission from his medical school to do a four-week rotation in my clinic. In order for him to get credit for the rotation, I had to give him a test, which he had to pass, at the end of his time with me.

I'm not a fan of testing. It rarely measures capability or capacity to think. I'd much prefer a kind of apprentice system in which an experienced practitioner knows a student well enough to somehow publicly state that the young doctor is ready to be on his own. But this young student needed a test in order to get the credit, so I gave him a test. Actually, I gave him both a pretest and posttest that had the same questions: Describe the physiological significance of the paintings by Raphael and van Dyck of

St. George slaying the dragon, and the physiological significance of Botticelli's *The Birth of Venus*. On the pretest, my student wrote that he had never heard of any of these paintings or even any of these artists. On the posttest, he gave a passable rendition of the significance of both paintings.

At this point, I would almost like people to pause, get and read Mark Booth's *New York Times*–best-selling book *The Secret History of the World*, and then resume reading this chapter. I will assume, however, that most of my readers won't do that, so I'll try to explain as best I can why I would ask this medical student such unusual questions. (Appendix B on page 167 contains what I believe to be the "correct" answers to the above questions, for those who are interested.) Through the course of history, certain people have been proponents of what is sometimes called the perennial philosophy. This philosophy describes a way of understanding the world around us, and the long course of human evolution. In particular, this philosophy is concerned with the evolution of human thought—more specifically, human consciousness—which has evolved over time just as our bodies have. As Booth so cogently explains, most historical leaders were initiated into an understanding of this philosophy and many claim its teachings inspired their great works. Raphael, van Dyck, and Botticelli were three of these initiates and openly referred to the esoteric origins of their masterpieces. In essence, they were depicting knowledge of the human being, in an artistic form, that served as a vital tool for human consciousness.

In our current educational model—and, medical education, in particular—there is no awareness of or appreciation for the history of esoteric thought. I don't believe anyone can be a true physician, however, without an understanding of Shakespeare's (another initiate) Hamlet and his struggle to understand the meaning of his own existence. In order to understand the lives and struggles of our patients, to understand the human condition in the fullest sense, we must be familiar with Dostoyevsky (another initiate) and his investigation into man's struggle with his own conscience. These inspired stories, and many others, weave the fabric of western culture.

If we, as doctors, are to be competent guides to people—often whose "poor" choices lead them into suffering and disease—we have to understand something of human consciousness and the human condition, and the masters of art and literature, from both eastern and western traditions, have so much to offer us in this regard. Sadly, even in psychiatry there is no reference to these seminal works in the history of the understanding of the human being. As George Orwell, another writer who credits his insight to the lessons he learned through his initiation, predicted in *1984*, we are becoming a people without a past, a crucial step in undermining our humanity. Yes, today's physicians can remove a sick gall bladder, or a cataract that's hindering a patient's vision. But that is mechanics, not healing. Modern medicine is not only unaware of where and how healing comes about, but is fundamentally antagonistic to even exploring the idea. This is deeply unfortunate for our patients, and for society at large.

Fundamentally, what I am suggesting is that the great esoteric traditions have a lot to teach us about unseen realities, including the nature of consciousness, the nature of wholeness, and the tension between health and disease.

For anyone who undertakes the study of these traditions, it is striking how much depth of understanding ancient teachings contain in them and what they can offer—personally, spiritually, intellectually—even for the most practical or mechanistically minded professions.

The core myths or allegories of both eastern and western culture give us a blueprint for understanding, down to the details, even a problem like cancer.

All philosophies are concerned with wholeness, the nature of being, the human condition, and helping people understand and make peace with the world we inhabit. The yin-yang symbol is one of the simplest and most enduring encapsulations of this.

It's not just about balance. It shows us that the world is created by the merging of two primal and opposite forces that, when joined together in a harmonious way, create health and wholeness. Furthermore, and paradoxically, both yin and yang contain a kernel of the opposite force in their essences, representing the healthy and necessary tension between the two.

Here is another way to think about health and harmony: The first book of the Old Testament, Genesis, is a creation story that begins with the separation of light from darkness. Combined, these two great forces comprise the totality of the universe and human existence. There is never complete darkness. We all know that the darkest time of night is right before the dawn. Even pitch darkness contains the seeds of the new light to come. We are being taught, through this essential story, that in order to understand the creation of the universe and the creation of consciousness, we have to look at the separation of these two forces as a primal event. In order to achieve harmony, health, or consciousness, these forces must coexist, in balance.

Of course, there is no one story or symbol to guide us. There are many. None is perhaps as powerful as the story of the birth of Jesus, offering yet another foundational myth. Western civilization wouldn't exist without the Judeo-Christian narrative that forms its philosophical and spiritual underpinnings. To be clear, I am not arguing for the correctness of the story of Jesus's birth. I am not interested in whether we believe the story to be literally accurate. I am suggesting that no matter your beliefs, the story of the birth of Jesus is, at least, an allegory for a turning point in the development of our civilization. If we look at this story as written in the Gospels, we find a strange tale. In the Gospel of Matthew, we learn that Jesus is a direct descendant of the line of the famous Hebrew King David. The precise lineage of his descent from King David, through Joseph, is outlined in great detail. In other words, we are given Jesus's specific lineage on his paternal side.

In the Gospel of Luke, however, there is no mention of paternal heritage. In fact, we are told that an angel informs the young virgin, Mary, that she is carrying the son of God. Mary replies that this is not possible since she is still a virgin, and we are told that "with God all things are possible." What are we to make of such contradictory stories? And what are we to make of the coexistence of this narrative with the yin-yang symbolism of eastern traditions? Both are so utterly foundational to mythology, history, and human consciousness. It is in that coexistence, that *tension*, where, I believe, we can begin to understand the etiology of cancer in a very different light than western medicine presents to us today.

If we take both narratives as attempts to provide a picture of creation and the forces that underlie the creation of the human being and the fostering of wholeness, we can find some immediate similarities. Both narrative traditions speak about wholeness as arising from the coexistence and merging of two opposites. The yin-yang symbol is the harmonious merger of the light and the dark. In the birth story of Jesus, the archetype of humanity (Jesus) arises from the merging of the hereditary, male side as represented by the lineage of Joseph, and the angelic, maternal side, as represented by Mary. As we read further into this story, we are instructed that the male force works through heredity, through individuals with real names, biographies, and historical lives on earth, whereas the female force comes from another realm entirely, via the annunciation from an angel. This story tells us that creation, and wholeness, comes from the merging of the material, earthly substance with forces that are not of this world, at least not in their origin. The next question is: What does this mean for, and where do we find this in, human physiology?

To understand the creation of a human being, we must go back to the beginning and examine the two cells that come together. Before there was any understanding of genetics, fertilization, or any of the tenets of modern biology, these stories arose from an understanding that a human being is created from the merger of two great forces. Remember that the yin-yang symbol tells us that darkness, or light, always contains a touch of its opposite force. We can characterize the sperm as a compressed package of DNA, representing the distilled nucleus of a cell, essentially a motorized packet of DNA containing just a touch of watery cytoplasm.

The egg, on the other hand, can be thought of as an expanded, and water-filled cytoplasm, so swollen with water that the egg is the only cell actually visible to the naked eye. The cytoplasm, as represented by Mary in the story of Jesus's birth, suggests a force not primarily concerned with heredity, which is downplayed almost to the point of nonexistence, with only a trace of hereditary material contained in the mitochondria. The mitochondria have their own set of DNA—it is the tiny bit of the DNA housed in the cytoplasm, represented in the yin-yang symbol—and are passed down through the maternal line. In other words, we inherit our mitochondria from our mother. The maternal line is the source of the cytoplasmic blueprint of her offspring.

The human being is created out of this merger of the dense, nuclear male side and the watery, maternal feminine side. As the Jesus story suggests, the male force determines the primary characteristics of a new human being, the most primary characteristic of all being its sex. To be more succinct, although this is only hinted at in these stories, the sperm or male force gives us our individual characteristics—again our sex being the most primary characteristic of all—whereas the egg, or female force, gives us the nonmaterial aspects of our being. The female force is more universal, less differentiated in its essence. Researchers using sophisticated microscopic techniques have been able to demonstrate that the traveling sperm emits a kind of luminescence as it seeks out its partner the egg. The egg lies in the darkness, the sperm emits light. When the sperm merges with the darkness of the egg, a new human being is formed.

Over the past two thousand years, there have been many stories of healing associated with the story of Jesus, and the preponderance of these involve some interaction with Mary, as the source of healings. The most famous story is of Mary blessing the waters in Lourdes, where approximately seven thousand miraculous healings have taken place, as documented and certified by the French government. Setting aside the argument of whether these accounts are verifiable or technically accurate—which I realize brews like a tempest in our mechanistic minds as I type these words—the stories of these healings often involve profound spiritual experiences and almost always involve the person of Mary (as opposed to Joseph) and, of course, water.

My suggestion is that the healing or therapeutic part of the Joseph–Mary polarity, or the nucleus–cytoplasm polarity, resides in the *cytoplasm, not the nucleus*. It is Mary, the watery cytoplasmic force, that has the primary power to heal human beings, and the planet as a whole. The nuclear side, though crucial in our evolution toward becoming free individuals, also leads us to disease.

I would expect—even hope at this point—that none of my readers will accept these statements at face value, though I hope you're at least willing to travel down the mental path with me. Furthermore, even if there are many unexplained stories of healings associated with Mary, or sacred waters, how do we know we're not just dealing with the immense power of belief, the placebo effect? A healthy amount of skepticism, if not outright cynicism, is in order here. I acknowledge that, and accept it. What I'm saying is that these stories give us a different framework to begin to think about health and disease—and cancer specifically—in a different way. It's a different framework of thinking, which I argue we need, because the current oncogene model, based on a mechanistic conception of the human body and genetic determinism, isn't working very well.

In fact, some research about the underlying dynamics of what causes cancer substantiates what I have laid out in an almost uncanny way. This is especially poignant since modern biology, modern medicine, and specifically modern oncology have put their focus, almost entirely, on understanding the events that happen in the *nucleus* of the cell. If my interpretation is correct, then the unfortunate implication is that we will never find that which can bring harmony and wholeness to our cancer patients because the location in which this healing is to be found is the cytoplasm, not the nucleus. I believe we have been looking in the wrong place. We have been desperately looking in the nucleus, at DNA, at oncogenes, as the watery cytoplasm lies in wait for us to realize that just because the nucleus contains more light, it doesn't mean that's where we should be looking to find our keys.

If we think back to the hypothetical carrot example, there is a clear difference (in our minds) between the physical substances that make up a carrot and what we call a carrot. One of the people who attempted to explore this difference was the renowned twentieth-century physicist Erwin Schrödinger. In his fascinating book, *What Is Life?*, Schrödinger attempts to use his considerable observational skills combined with his expertise in theoretical physics to give a definition and working model of the question, "What is life?"[1] As Schrödinger reminds us, material objects are subject to many forces, including gravity and entropy. Gravity, we all know about: Things tend to fall toward the center of earth unless acted upon by levity. Entropy is not so well known, but is as fundamental as gravity. Entropy relates to the degree of order or disorder acting upon material objects.

Simply put, material objects always fall toward the center of the earth (gravity) and tend toward a progressively disordered state unless acted upon by an external force. Take, for example, a handful of completely dry sand (a good approximation of a totally physical substance). If no other forces act on it, the sand will fall and its form will be an indistinct heap on the ground. This is the state substances assume unless acted on by external forces. In physics this is referred to as the state of maximum entropy. According to Schrödinger, however, *life* is characterized by an opposite force, for which he coined a new word—*negentropy*, the opposite of entropy.

Before we go any further, first a note of caution: When we discuss life and negentropy, or what Rudolf Steiner referred to as the etheric body, we need to remember that our language hasn't evolved sufficiently to allow us to easily describe what we're talking about; our language privileges events in the physical world. Consequently, a lot of people shy away from attempting to describe or even talk about such things. This is a mistake. We need to acknowledge that while language is an imperfect tool, making it challenging to be precise and communicate effectively, that doesn't mean language isn't where the keys are to be found. It means we need to keep trying, and keep looking.

Going back to our carrot and taking cues from Schrödinger, we can make a few simple observations: When trying to describe the phenomena of life, it is simplest to start with "simpler" life-forms, such as plants, rather than trying to describe an elephant or a human being. (Plants aren't simple, but according to Goethe and Steiner, they are simpler and more rewarding to study when asking the question "What is life?") The first thing we notice about the carrot, as opposed to the heap of chemicals that make up the carrot, is that the carrot has a form that clearly identifies it as a carrot. The second observation is that the carrot has qualities, which not only identify it as a carrot but also give it value to us. The form of the carrot seems to defy both gravity and entropy. We know that to "defy" either gravity, entropy, or both, a substance must be acted upon by an external force. Here the language becomes tricky, but we can conclude that a carrot is the result of interplay between the substances making up the carrot and the force of levity, as well as negentropy, the tendency toward greater order. The next thing we notice is that in order for these two forces to influence the substances making up the carrot, water must be present. Without water, neither levity nor negentropy has any influence on the substance of the carrot. In other words, water is the necessary "carrier" of the two forces that comprise the essence of life.

All the properties of the carrot that we call the quality of the carrot arise as a result of the forces of levity and negentropy working through the water in the carrot. Just this morning I went on a long walk on the beach with my wife Lynda. I was trying to understand in my mind how to explain this idea of quality. What interested both of us is that even though it's a very difficult concept to describe, almost everyone has an immediate grasp of the existence of qualities as well as their importance. If we had to choose between a handmade table made by a local artisan out of locally sourced wood and a similar-looking, similarly priced factory-made table, almost everyone would choose the first. Why? The first is better quality. Quality in this sense doesn't only have to do with value, but also it has to do with the characteristics, or qualities, of the object.

What about two carrots? Let's say these carrots contain the same amount of nutrients (which we all know is never really the case) and look more or less the same. But one was grown on a small, sustainable biodynamic farm and the other was grown on an industrial farm in the Central Valley. Almost everyone will choose the biodynamic carrot. The only reason people give for not choosing quality in just about anything is the cost. Cost aside, a factor not intrinsic to a given object, human beings tend to spend their lives seeking out the highest quality of everything—goods, experiences, and so forth—they can reasonably obtain. My contention is that quality is a function of levity and negentropy, which is what enlivens something. Even the handmade table gets its value because of the presence of these forces in the wood that makes up the table and the craftsman who made it.

The next step in Schrödinger's investigation into the question of "What is life?" is his claim that entropy directly gives rise to the experience and reality of time. In other words, if entropy didn't exist as a governing principle of the physical world, neither would time. He goes on to offer mathematical proof. To be clear, I'm not in a position to assess whether he is correct, nor can I evaluate the mathematics underlying his proof. What I can do, however, is understand that, as he claims, if entropy "creates" the phenomena of time, then negentropy, which is the basis of life, is somehow a timeless state. Furthermore, this brings up the possibility that a living entity with an extremely robust force of levity and negentropy should be able to live as if there was no effect of time on its being. While this seems like an impossibility, we could conjecture that certain types of trees are the virtual embodiment of these negentropic/levity forces; as long as their natural habitat is undisturbed they can live thousands of years, maybe more. It's as if certain trees see time for what it is, an illusion created only because all life on earth is also composed of physical substance. And it is only the physical substance of living beings that is subject to the laws of time. The rest of "us," the living part of us, is not subject to the experience of time. One can hardly emphasize enough the significance of this possibility. What he is saying is that all living beings are living because they contain "within" themselves these forces of levity and negentropy. These forces give rise to the qualities that we associate with that unique living entity; they are what actually define the quality of that living organism. And, if one examines this situation closely, one finds that the laws governing time either do not apply to living beings or apply differently to living beings than to physical, nonliving substance. Perhaps this is the essence of the core of the Hindu philosophy, which claims that our experience of time is fundamentally an illusion.

The question then is: How does understanding these life forces that work through water and give rise to quality in living beings relate to either cancer or cell biology? Going back to our previous discussion of the two realms of the cell—the nucleus as represented by the almost totally desiccated sperm, and the watery realm of the egg—it is easy to see that the cytoplasm/egg domain must be the carrier of this principle of levity/negentropy. When this watery, cytoplasmic realm is "weak," disordered or hindered in some way, then we will see a dysfunction and disease arise. This will especially give rise to problems in our health that are specifically related to cytoplasmic function, such as cancer. This might include the failure of the cytoplasmic structures such as the mitochondria. When the mitochondria function poorly, energy generation is affected and the characteristics we noted about the cancer cell arise. Let's state this more succinctly: When our life forces are weak or disturbed, when the structure of water in our cells is amiss, the disease we call cancer arises. Therefore, the integrity of the water in our cells and the ways in which the water in our cells are structured or formed from these forces of levity and negentropy should be of utmost concern in addressing the problem of cancer.

Finally, if Schrödinger is correct in claiming that time results from entropy and this water/negentropic force counteracts the basic phenomena of time, then it should be possible, at least in theory, to strengthen these forces and reverse time in a living being. If this could be done on a cellular level, it should be possible to take a cell that has "degenerated" into a new and inappropriate "species" (that is, the aneuploid cell that is the cancer cell) and reverse this process and allow it to revert to a normal, healthy cell. As I said, I can't evaluate the correctness of the connection between time and entropy but I can evaluate whether a therapy that attempts to heal the "water" body can essentially reverse time for a patient with cancer and bring them "back" to a healthy state. That, after all, is what this discussion is all about.

In part two, I will examine some of the most significant and successful natural therapies used for cancer in the past century and their effectiveness in healing the water body. Some therapies, such as deuterium-depleted water, work with water directly. Others, such as mistletoe, help structure the water in our cells and tissues. Yet others impact the Na+/K+ balance. I will provide case studies and research results, and evaluate claims of effectiveness. In most cases, I have personal experience with these therapies and can speak directly to their safety and effectiveness. By describing these therapies from the perspective of their impact on the water body, we will hopefully gain a better understanding of the role of water in living organisms, which will in turn bring us closer to answering the riddle of the etiology of and therapy for cancer. Along with this, my hope is it brings us even closer to the understanding of what life is. To me, these therapies collectively represent a different path forward in addressing the epidemic problem of cancer in the western world.

Because I have written extensively elsewhere about prevention, particularly the impact of environmental toxicity, diet, the role of fever suppression, vaccines, electric and magnetic field exposure, and many other lifestyle factors, I won't spend a lot of time on prevention per se. My hope is that by focusing on successful treatment strategies and those that merit further exploration, it will also light the way to prevention. While I hope it goes without saying that prevention of cancer, or any disease, should be paramount, we are also currently in a situation where millions of our people and their families are facing the devastation of a diagnosis. This is despite more than fifty years of research, billions of dollars spent, and many of the best scientists in the world attempting to solve the riddle. We are seemingly not much further along in the quest to eradicate cancer than we were fifty years ago. In some ways, things are worse.

To be clear, I don't have a "this is the cure for cancer" formula to present in part two. Rather, I will present what I have learned from having practiced medicine for almost four decades. In that time, I have had personal experience with most of the significant "alternative" cancer programs available to people today, I have used most of them with my patients, and I know their strengths and weaknesses. For many of these therapies, I will present cases showing that they can help their users have longer, healthier lives. In other cases, I have seen dramatic, almost shocking, durable remissions.

Unfortunately, none of these cancer strategies are as reliably effective as we would all hope. I believe that one of the reasons this is so is that, as I will demonstrate, each, in its own way, addresses the understanding of cancer as a cytoplasmic disease without actually having the full picture. In many cases, even the originator or founder of the therapy did not know this was the issue he was addressing. I hope to demonstrate that whether the discoverer was aware of it or not, each was working directly with some aspect of this cytoplasmic dysfunction.

One of my reasons for writing this book is my hope that if we examine which therapies have actually worked, from the cytoplasmic perspective, in treating cancer patients, we can begin to not only understand the disease more fully, but also be able to consciously map out an effective strategy for far more people. Another reason I'm writing this book is to point out the remarkable fact that the amount of resources and money devoted to studying the entirety of these "alternative" therapies I will discuss is far less than 0.01 percent of the total resources devoted to cancer research. Yet one can argue that patients using the Gerson diet, mistletoe therapy, deuterium-depleted water, the Rife machine, or even those who take turmeric, have better outcomes than those patients who follow the standard of care.

Imagine what would have happened if in 1920, when some of the strategies I'm presenting in part two were first introduced, the power brokers in medicine had decided to spend 50 percent, or even 10 percent, of their resources looking into the natural approaches to the prevention and treatment of cancer. Would we have effective dietary and other natural, safe, effective approaches to the treatment of cancer patients by now? What might have happened if we had devoted *half* of our cancer budget to lifestyle, diet, agriculture—if we had, say, promoted organics instead of toxic agriculture eighty years ago—and other strategies to prevent a cancer epidemic in the first place.

Instead, the powers that be have exerted enormous effort and pressure to suppress these approaches. This has included direct personal attacks on proponents of natural therapies and the passage of laws that prohibit physicians from treating their cancer patients with anything other than the standard oncology approaches. In fact, in 2018, in the ostensibly progressive state of California, it was illegal for any licensed physician to prescribe anything besides chemotherapy, radiation, or surgery for a cancer patient. If a physician fails to comply, she risks losing her license and facing other possibly harsher penalties. Is this what we mean by the "land of the free"?

My hope is that by presenting the history of and rationale for the most successful natural approaches to cancer treatment we can begin to see the similarities they share. The inspiring stories of patients who have had success with these therapies will help us understand, if nothing else, that after a fifty-plus-year monopoly on the resources devoted to the understanding and treatment of cancer, the scientific and medical establishment no longer deserves its free pass. I'm not saying we should bulldoze all our cancer institutions to the ground, only that we should consider what a popular bumper sticker suggests: What would the world be like if the peace, justice, and environmental safety initiatives got all the resources they needed and the Pentagon had to hold bake sales to stay in business? It's time for conventional oncology departments to hold a few bake sales and for alternative treatment approaches—especially those that take a far less militaristic view of the human body and human health—to receive respectable funding.

Before we launch into the therapies, I would like to share the story of a young patient I have known for years. After a few months of knee pain, she was diagnosed with a malignant osteosarcoma around the left knee that had spread to her lungs. She was quickly seen and evaluated by world-renowned oncologists at Stanford University Medical Center, who mapped out her course of therapy. Like most oncologists, they had no knowledge of Coley's toxins, a successful fever therapy that was specifically used to treat osteosarcoma in the early twentieth century,[2] and gave her the standard of care treatment, which consists of a chemotherapy drug that has been around since the 1950s, followed by partial amputation of her leg.

As of this writing, it is too soon to tell whether her treatment will be effective, but we do know that the outcomes for sarcoma patients with metastatic disease are not good with standard of care treatment. The question is this: After fifty years of the most costly and extensive research ever undertaken on a given disease, why aren't we shocked and astounded that oncology seems to have nothing better, or even different, to offer than what was offered more than four or five decades ago? This is not like strep throat, for which penicillin has worked for almost a century (a qualified "work" to be sure). Standard of care has been a largely unsuccessful approach for many decades. So why do we prohibit anyone from trying something different, especially when the something different was less harmful and possibly more success-ful? Why has Coley's toxins, which was developed *specifically* to treat osteosarcoma, never been investigated by our oncology establishment? Nobody knows if it would work because investi-gating it has been forbidden.

The geneticist who saw this young woman to explain the "genetics" and "cause" of her cancer explained that tumors and cancers are caused by uncontrolled cell growth and proliferation due to genetic disruption of cell cycle regulation. There are many genes in the human body that are important for controlling cell growth and preventing cancer, which is caused by mutations or differences in the genetic sequence of one of these genes. But, the geneticist went on to explain, in most cases the cause of sar-coma is unknown, and it is considered an isolated, sporadic occurrence of unknown etiology.

In other words, though according to this geneticist cancer is a genetic disease, we have no clue how or why you get it. You may have no family history of the disease, there are no known genetic mutations that we can find, there is no clear evidence that sarcomas are associated with any particular genetic defect—we just don't know. Fifty years, billions of dollars, and a network of researchers studying this issue more intensively than any other issue has ever been studied in the history of mankind, and we have nothing for you. Just take this drug that stops cells from dividing and we'll partially amputate your leg and hope for the best. Just whatever you do, don't investigate or try any "unproven" approaches. That would not be safe.

With that said, let's turn our attention to some of these "unproven" approaches to see what they might yield.

PART II

Potential Therapies

CHAPTER FOUR

Quinton Isotonic Plasma

The 1925 death of French physiologist René Quinton prompted one of the largest funeral processions in the history of France. The thousands of people attending it lined the streets, heads of state flocked in, and the prime minister of France delivered the eulogy for a man most of us have never heard of but whose life work saved untold numbers of lives at the time, formed a cornerstone of modern medical practice, and offers practical insight that belongs at the center of any attempt to understand the role of structured water in health and disease.

Who was René Quinton? What did he accomplish that led to this outpouring of admiration and support? He was a humble man who worked with seawater his entire adult life. He is credited with the development of a rehydration solution that saved the lives of many people, mostly children, who were dying of cholera in French cities during the early twentieth century. Quinton plasma, as it would come to be known, was also used by the French military to resuscitate soldiers wounded in the battles of the First World War, and was so effective that the French government established Quinton centers throughout the country to treat people, often children, for many different illnesses.

Of course, it also became the blueprint that gave rise to the intravenous (IV) solutions used in modern medicine, as well as the oral rehydration solutions used, for example, by the World Health Organization to combat dehydration from diarrhea that is still such a menace to residents of the global south or those living in areas hit by natural disasters. Inevitably, the quality of modern IV fluids is a shell of Quinton's original development. Whereas modern IV fluids are now just sodium chloride in sterile water packaged into plastic bags, Quinton, having observed that our blood and extracellular fluids (the fluids in which our cells are bathed) have the same mineral composition as seawater, created a plasma composed of seawater.

Quinton's discovery that our blood reflects the mineral composition of the oceans led him to propose the idea that health can be defined as the state in which our fluids, including blood, are in their "perfect" state when they most closely mirror the composition of the sea. Disease, according to Quinton, arises when this internal mineral balance is disturbed. Furthermore, he proposed that the internal fluids are not just a suspension of a particular mix of minerals and water but exist in a kind of organized state. This organized state is another aspect of the health of the organism. When our internal fluids are in perfect mineral balance, in their optimal organized state, we are healthy. When the mineral composition is off or the organization breaks down, we suffer disease.

Quinton was not content to propose abstract theories about the nature of health and disease, however. He reasoned that if he was correct, then the proper application of seawater should be able to restore a sick person to health. Over decades of research he discovered that there are a few areas of the oceans with, for unexplained reasons, permanent natural vortexes several miles wide. Within these vortexes are (of course) seawater, phytoplankton, and other microscopic sea organisms. Quinton and his colleagues developed techniques to drop a suction apparatus deep within the center of this nutrient-rich vortex and essentially suck the seawater out of the vortex into large tanks. (In my book *Human Heart, Cosmic Heart*, I proposed that circulation arises from forces intrinsic to the blood itself and that the role of the heart is to convert this movement of the blood into a vortex to imbue it with the "creative energy" that is the basis of all life. Quinton, with his technique of collecting seawater containing the mineral composition of human blood from a nutrient-rich vortex, was essentially re-creating the heart's role in a human being.)

Quinton knew that this vortexed seawater needed to be microfiltered before use and that the purification technique had to preserve the delicate structure of the water that was created by the vortexing. He did this by developing a series of filters that eliminated everything but the water, the dissolved minerals, and the dissolved "effluent" of the phytoplankton. These two aspects—the harvesting of the seawater from deep in the ocean vortexes and the cold, microfiltration of the resulting water—distinguish Quinton plasma from all the other seawater solutions that have ever been produced or sold. Quinton was not, as some have claimed, just collecting a bunch of seawater and putting it in bottles. He was collecting and purifying what was probably the best example of properly structured water we know of.

The components of structured water in any living system are pure water (more on this in subsequent chapters), the proper mineral elements (those found in a healthy ocean), and proteins (coming from the phytoplankton in the ocean)—put through a vortex. Quinton plasma has all of these components, all meticulously and properly collected and cared for.

Quinton's basic idea was that purified, mineralized, nutrient-rich, structured water is the basis of all biological life. To prove this, he conducted laboratory experiments in which he drained nearly all the blood out of a sick dog. Right before the dog expired, he started a drip of Quinton plasma into the dog's veins. The dog not only survived but was cured of many of the ailments it was suffering from. Quinton and his colleagues did this same demonstration in the center of Paris to show people the power of the discovery he had made. Many remarked that the dogs who had their blood replaced with Quinton plasma looked and acted years younger than before this dramatic procedure.

Today, Quinton plasma is not known as a cancer therapy per se, and I haven't encountered any case reports or studies showing effectiveness with cancer patients solely from the use of Quinton plasma, but I firmly believe it belongs in any treatise that attempts to understand the role of structured or cytoplasmic water in health and disease, which is what I think our understanding of cancer must revolve around. Pure, mineralized, nutrient-rich, structured water is the biological basis for all life. When our internal fluids are degraded, whether by toxins, infection, even harmful emotions, disease ensues. The Quinton Foundation was established in 2010 to further the work and therapies of René Quinton and catalogs various conditions that can be treated by Quinton therapy as well as protocols for successful treatment. In the past few decades, independent studies have documented the safety and efficacy of Quinton plasma to treat conditions including influenza,[1] hypertension,[2] Alzheimer's disease,[3] immune dysfunction,[4] diabetes,[5] obesity,[6] progression of atherosclerosis,[7] hyperlipidemia,[8] and allergic rhinitis.[9]

While modern medical practitioners may find it hard to imagine that a single therapy could positively affect such a disparate collection of maladies, that is because they are still stuck in the individual disease model of health and disease. My premise, like René Quinton's, is that if we are able to create the perfect structured water in and around our cells, we will be immune to most disease. If we are sick, we need to reestablish this more perfect cytoplasmic, cellular milieu. Quinton plasma was one of the most successful and creative attempts to accomplish just this goal.

Thanks to the Quinton Foundation, Quinton's original "recipe" is still available, and for the last few years plasma based on this recipe has been available for use by people in the United States (see appendix A, page 165). I consider Quinton plasma, along with a proper diet, to be one of the foundations of my practice. My family members and I have taken a couple table-spoons of Quinton plasma nearly every day for the past number of years. I can think of no reason why every person who is concerned about either maintaining or improving their health shouldn't take Quinton plasma every day. It has an unblemished safety record of over a hundred years, is the most effective mineral supplement on the planet, and demonstrably improves the cellular milieu for all its users. I see no reason why, with such a safe, effective, and reasoned biological approach, more studies of this marvelous medicine shouldn't be done.

CHAPTER FIVE

Gerson Therapy

When I was twenty years old, newly graduated from Duke University, and setting off for a stint in the Peace Corps in Swaziland, Africa, I had no idea what I wanted to do with my life. The only thing I knew for sure was that I didn't want to be a doctor. Over the course of two years living in a mud-walled, grass-roofed hut in rural Swaziland, I encountered the work of Weston Price and Rudolf Steiner. It was a revelation to realize that the type of doctor I had vowed never to be was not the only type of doctor there is. It was as if a dam burst and I found myself reading and studying this new type of medicine with a fervor I'd never expected nor experienced. I couldn't learn enough about food, herbs, anthroposophy, and the amazing world of healing and healers fast enough.

When I returned from the Peace Corps I enrolled in Michigan State's medical school, and continued my pursuit of natural healing theories and methods. I also joined a newly formed group called the Physicians' Association for Anthroposophical Medicine (PAAM), a branch of the global anthroposophical medicine movement. I attended a week-long conference every year in Wilton, New Hampshire, read everything I could get my hands on, and attended every relevant workshop and lecture I could find. In 1983, during my third year in medical school, I got permission to do all my electives with the small group of practicing anthroposophical doctors in various centers in the eastern United States.

In 1983, I attended a lecture given by a young doctor about his healing journey. He had recently finished his family practice residency and was serving as president of PAAM. In the lecture, he shared the story of his journey from metastatic testicular cancer, rejecting conventional oncology treatments, embarking on the Gerson therapy, and his subsequent total remission a few years later. During the workshop, he went into the details of his diagnosis, leaving no doubt that he was, in fact, dealing with stage 4 testicular cancer. He outlined the details of his therapy, and read statements from his oncologists saying that he would soon die if he didn't submit to conventional medicine. Finally he spoke about his full recovery, complete with the tests and scans documenting the absence of cancer. To say I was intrigued and impressed is to put it mildly.

I read everything I could find about the Gerson diet, including Max Gerson's famous book *Cancer Therapy: Results of Fifty Cases*, in which he outlines the development of his thinking, the rationale for his therapy, and then the documentation of fifty cured cases that he compiled and presented to the US Congress in the late 1940s. At that time, a Senate subcommittee was conducting hearings on the type of cancer research and treatments it was going to fund. Gerson presented his cases with in-person testimonials by patients who'd been cured after following his therapy, including X-rays and blood tests to document the veracity of his claims. (In an interesting historical footnote, the hearings on cancer funding ended with a very close vote in favor of the chemical, chemotherapeutic approach of the major pharmaceutical interests as opposed to the more natural, nutritional approaches advocated by Max Gerson and others. I sometimes wonder how much this turning point led us to the dreadful situation we currently find ourselves in—and how it might have gone differently.)

Max Gerson was a German-born physician who fled Nazi Germany and then worked alongside his friend Albert Schweitzer in Africa before moving to the United States. Gerson's primary interest early in his career was the development of a successful dietary approach to the treatment of tuberculosis. Eventually his "fat-free" dietary approach became widely used in European tuberculosis treatment centers, and he became fairly well known for this. After moving to the United States, he turned his attention to cancer and used many of the same principles he found successful in the treatment of tuberculosis. Gerson therapy is often interpreted as a detoxification program based on a vegan diet, vegetable juices, and coffee enemas, but that isn't an accurate interpretation of the therapy and doesn't reflect Gerson's rationale for its effectiveness.

Gerson thought that the foundation of disease was a disruption in the proper sodium-potassium gradient between the inside and the outside of the cell, such that cells begin to accumulate sodium and disease follows. According to Gerson, disease follows because a cell without this healthy sodium-potassium gradient is an uncharged, and therefore dead, cell, so every component of his therapy was based on the restoration of this sodium-potassium gradient.

Not long after Gerson started applying his therapy to cancer, in 1957, Danish scientist Jens Christian Skou discovered a sodium-potassium pump embedded in the cell membrane that most mainstream scientists believe is responsible for ferrying sodium out of the cell and potassium into it, helping to explain how mammalian cells live in a sodium-rich milieu, yet maintain a low sodium state inside their cells.[1] Dr. Gilbert Ling subsequently showed the fallacy of this pump—not that it exists (it does), but that its role is misplaced, misunderstood, and overstated in mainstream science—but the significance of the sodium-potassium gradient itself cannot be overstated. Besides *Digitalis* (which I will discuss in chapter 6), there was, at the time of Skou's discovery, no practical way to work with this sodium-potassium pump to effect the sodium-potassium balance. Gerson had the sense that if he could affect this balance, he could radically change the energetics of the cell and thereby reduce the likelihood of disease.

Gerson therefore conceived of a diet based on increasing potassium and dramatically reducing sodium. No salt of any type was permitted on the diet. At times, he even excluded celery because it's a fairly unique plant in that it tends to accumulate sodium. Most animal foods were excluded not because Gerson believed in the healing power of a vegan diet—as is commonly misinterpreted today—but because animal foods tend to be higher in sodium than plant foods. In fact, Gerson insisted on fresh raw liver juice every two hours during the intensive phase of his program and included high doses of animal thyroid, which he said stimulated the sodium-potassium balance and helped drive the sodium out of the cells and the potassium back into the cells. Gerson was able to demonstrate that with time this extraordinarily high potassium intake coupled with almost no sodium did, in fact, change the sodium-potassium gradient across the cell membrane.

Gerson also insisted that his patients use a specific grind-and-press juicer, the Norwalk Juicer, which he helped the manufacturer develop, to make the carrot, beet, apple, and liver juice patients needed to consume in large quantities every day. These days, we talk about juicing as a way to detox, but that wasn't Gerson's original intent. The Norwalk Juicer is the only juicer that left the energy structure of the intracellular component with its "attached" potassium intact enough from the juiced vegetables to be taken up by the cells of his patients. We know now that the intracellular component of a carrot, beet, or apple is structured water, which retains the potassium in its matrix. Like Quinton's plasma (but without using vortexes), Gerson's therapy took advantage of the natural tendency of all living things to structure their intracellular space. Gerson's goal was to try to extract this intracellular, cytoplasmic component intact enough to be taken up and utilized by the sick patient.

When I learned about Gerson therapy, I was so impressed by the results that I might be the only physician in the United States who asked his parents for a Norwalk Juicer as a graduation present from medical school. Gerson was adamant that Gerson therapy without a Norwalk Juicer was a recipe for failure. The juicers are very expensive and my hope was that if I had one, I could loan it out to my patients as they began their own Gerson therapy. After about thirty-five years, I still have it, it still works, and I still use it to make juice and other tinctures and foods. Over the years, I have probably consumed thousands of glasses of Norwalk Juicer–made carrot juice and loaned my juicer out to scores of patients.

Another integral component of Gerson's therapy was his soup made mostly from plant roots with some other vegetables mixed in. The plants were chosen because of their high potassium content and making them into a broth was a way to get access to proteins that are used as scaffolding for the intracellular matrix, so the broth was another method for increasing the intracellular potassium and structuring the intracellular water. This is similar to other well-known cancer therapies that use large doses of collagen, such as Dr. John Prudden's cartilage therapy or shark cartilage treatments. These are all variations on the theme of creating healthier intracellular structured water.

Gerson did include coffee enemas as an aid in detoxification to dilate the bile ducts, helping the liver clear toxins through the intestines more efficiently. But even this basic detoxification strategy was thought to help restore the sodium-potassium balance by clearing out toxins that had accumulated in the intracellular space. One of the primary ways that our intracellular gels get distorted is by the introduction of toxins that get absorbed into the cells. These toxins then bind with the gel, distorting its structure. Distorted gels are not the proper configuration to exclude sodium or bind potassium. As a result, the exclusion of sodium is lessened, the charge across the membrane is weakened, and the cell loses its charge and therefore its energy. The cells without charges clump together into a tumor. Eliminating the accumulated toxins in the cells through techniques such as coffee enemas helps to reverse this slide into worsening disease.

There are other minor components of the Gerson therapy, which is now used worldwide in the treatment of cancer patients. All of these components, when properly understood, facilitate this mineral gradient and charge production in the cells. The Gerson diet should not be marketed as a vegan or even vegetarian diet; it never was either of these. It should not be used as a rationale for why humans should adopt vegan diets unless eating large quantities of fresh liver can be considered an integral part of a vegan diet. The Gerson program was a brilliant and innovative approach to the restoration of the sodium-potassium balance across the cell membrane. There were even published studies showing how Gerson therapy was an innovative way to apply the principles discussed by Dr. Ling in his important works on the role of sodium-potassium balance in human health and disease.[2] Unfortunately, because this role was never properly understood, even by Gerson himself, the therapy falls short of being the final solution to the problem of cancer.

Over the years, it has saddened me to see people undertake what is unquestionably an arduous approach to the treatment of cancer, with its every-two-hour coffee enemas and copious intake of freshly made juice, only to fail to have the results we hoped for. There is no doubt that many people have been helped by Gerson therapy. Studies confirm this.[3] Documentaries show the stories of successful Gerson therapy cases. Yet many cases end similarly to the case of my friend with testicular cancer: After about a decade the cancer returned, and he simply didn't have the stomach to retry the Gerson therapy. He chose conventional chemotherapy at that time and fairly quickly died of the disease.

Gerson therapy should take its place in the annals of successful approaches to cancer therapy. It has much to teach us about how to approach patients with cancer, but in my view, because Gerson lacked a full understanding of the dynamics of intracellular gels and the role of the cytoplasm in the creation of disease, his therapy was destined to not be the final word on the quest for the successful treatment of a cancer patient.

CHAPTER SIX

Cardiac Glycosides

I n the mid-1990s, before I knew anything about the problems with sodium-potassium pump theory, I stumbled on research showing that cancer patients who took *Digitalis* preparations had better outcomes than those who did not. *Digitalis*, otherwise known as foxglove, has been used for treating cardiac arrhythmias and congestive heart failure for centuries. Its leaves are known to contain two active ingredients, digoxin and digitoxin, and originally the medicine was simply a preparation of dried *Digitalis* leaves. Both digoxin and digitoxin inhibit the activity of the sodium-potassium pump by binding to one of its protein components, leading to an influx of calcium into the cells, particularly cardiac cells. Calcium stimulates muscle contraction, so this leads to an improvement in the contractile force that the heart is able to generate, known as an inotropic effect. This improvement in the force of contraction is the reason that *Digitalis* was, for centuries, the central treatment for congestive heart failure, which was thought to be due to weak contractile force generated by the heart.

As time went on, other plant extracts were identified that affect the sodium-potassium pump, increasing the inotropic (contraction) ability of the heart. These include g-strophanthin, also known as ouabain, which is isolated from the *Strophanthus gratus* plant; bufolin, which is obtained from the skin of toads (and possibly the origin of the fairy tales revolving around kissing toads); and oleadrine, isolated from the oleander plant. As is usually the case, as more research was done on these various cardiac glycosides, the story became more complex.

It turns out that the various glycosides have different properties. For example, g-strophanthin is water-soluble, whereas digoxin is fat-soluble. Different glycosides also have different effects on the sodium-potassium balance, and in some cases the effect is dose dependent. For example, low doses of g-strophanthin stimulate the sodium-potassium pump, whereas high doses inhibit this pump. This also may be true for *Digitalis* glycosides; digoxin and digitoxin themselves may have slightly different biological effects from each other.

Gerson's work showed that cancer is related to, if not caused by, imbalances in this sodium-potassium gradient and that rebalancing it can have an impact on cancer outcomes, so it would stand to follow that medication that could restore this balance could positively impact a patient with cancer. In other words, if there were a medicine that stimulated an improvement in the sodium-potassium gradient across the cell membrane, thereby restoring the charge in the cell, it would be like Gerson therapy in pill form. In the 1990s, in fact, research was conducted that showed that *Digitalis* or g-strophanthin at appropriate doses can restore the sodium-potassium balance and lead to improvement in cancer outcomes. A 1999 study published in *Oncology Reports* stated, "The present study is a long-term follow-up (22.3 years) of 175 patients with breast carcinoma, of which 32 were on digitalis treatment when they acquired their breast cancer. There was a lower death rate (6%) from breast carcinoma among these patients on digitalis, when compared with patients not on digitalis (34%)."[1]

Other studies examined the mechanism whereby *Digitalis* affects cancerous growth. A 1999 study published in *Medical*

Hypotheses noted the ability of *Digitalis* to block cell proliferation, including apoptosis (cell death) in different malignant cell lines.[2] A 2009 study in the *American Journal of the Medical Sciences* reached a similar conclusion—that *Digitalis* inhibits cell growth and induces apoptosis in multiple cell cancer lines. "It is reasonable to expect," the article notes, "that the addition of digitalis to current cancer treatments will improve the clinical outcomes."[3] And a 2006 article in *Breast Cancer Research and Treatment* established that "there are several lines of evidence indicating that ouabain and related digitalis . . . possess potent anti-breast cancer activity" and called it "a new paradigm for development of anti-breast cancer drugs."[4]

The theme of this research is that cardiac glycosides, in particular digitoxin and g-strophanthin, at appropriate doses have a strong stimulation effect on the sodium-potassium pump, thereby restoring the healthy sodium-potassium distribution across the cell membrane, which then restores the charge and function of the cell. This is exactly what Gerson was trying to accomplish with his intensive therapy.

Armed with this insight in the 1990s, I set out to get access to preparations of *Digitalis* leaves or *Strophanthus* seeds to help my cancer patients, but a number of things made this search difficult. It was clear, for example, from the literature and the history, that *Digitalis* preparations made from the leaves of the *Digitalis* plant worked better and were less toxic than synthetically produced digoxin, which was the only *Digitalis* medicine available at the time. The same was true for *Strophanthus*, which worked better and was safer than using isolated chemically produced g-strophanthin, as it seems there are necessary synergistic components in the seeds, without which g-strophanthin is ineffective. After a lot of false starts, I eventually found an herbalist who would grow or wildcraft *Digitalis* and make it into a tincture. I had it tested to confirm that both digoxin and digitoxin were present in the tincture and then gave it to many of my patients with prostate cancer, since that was the cancer that seemed to have the best results from taking *Digitalis* preparations.

I observed that *Digitalis* extract definitely helped keep cancer from progressing, recurring, or growing as quickly. The patients who took the *Digitalis* extract consistently claimed that they felt better and had more energy, and that—even if they still had cancer—their quality of life was improved. In no cases, however, did I see a significant reduction in the size of their tumors or a significant lowering of the prostate-specific antigen (PSA), a blood marker for prostate cancer. My conclusion was that *Digitalis* was helpful but not dramatically so.

Since *Digitalis* can be toxic at too high a dose, I started every patient on a low dose and told them they had to get a blood test exactly one week after starting the medicine. As happens in medical practice, while most people are pretty good at following instructions, inevitably some people never seem to get it right. On at least five occasions, patients had their blood drawn *before* starting the extract. When I called them after receiving the test results and told them their blood levels were too low and they should increase the dose, they replied that they hadn't started taking the drops yet because they were waiting for the test results. What surprised me is that while the levels were indeed low, in all five cases there were testable levels of both digoxin and digitoxin in their blood even though they had never taken a single drop of any *Digitalis* preparation at any time in their lives. How could this be?

It turns out that digoxin, digitoxin, and g-strophanthin are naturally occurring compounds made in our adrenal cortex, seeming to regulate the sodium-potassium balance of the heart cells. The *Digitalis* and *Strophanthus* plants essentially make bioidentical copies of these endogenously produced hormones, which can be used as a medicine to augment the effect. This is similar to giving someone thyroid hormones when their own thyroid is not producing enough on its own.

My journey through the world of cardiac glycosides was full of such surprises. In the late 1990s, I received an email from a Brazilian man who asked me if my cancer patients on *Digitalis* extract suffered fewer heart attacks than I would otherwise expect. This struck me as an odd question, particularly because there was no reason to think that just because they had prostate cancer they would also have heart disease. At that time, I didn't know of any connection between *Digitalis* and heart attacks. Investigating this connection directly led to my later writings about the cause of heart attacks and their relation to cardiac glycosides, in particular *Strophanthus*.[5]

Soon after this fortuitous email, I learned about the work of Dr. Gilbert Ling, who critiqued the sodium-potassium pump theory and argued that the distribution of sodium and potassium across the cell wall is, in fact, a result of the configuration of the structured water in the intracellular space, which, when healthy, gives the cytoplasm its gel consistency and structure. He stated that this gel structure can exist in various phases or configurations and that changes in the phase or configuration allow the cell to accomplish various tasks. The best way to picture this is to imagine a window blind. In one configuration, the blind is shut and little light enters the room. Then by twisting the wand, the configuration shifts and light floods the room. One simple twist impacts all of the slats that make up the blind.

Similarly, the gels in our cells can exist in various phases or configurations. The addition of a few molecules triggers an almost instantaneous change in phase or configuration of the entire intracellular gel. This change then causes other changes to take place. New proteins are built, new parts of the DNA are expressed, muscles contract or relax. As with blinds, you don't need to change every water molecule in the cell; you just need to trigger the control mechanism and the rest cascades.

Ling went on to say that there are a very few "cardinal absorbents," which is what he called the substances a cell uses to trigger these phase changes. One such substance he found was ouabain, the cardiac glycoside I have written extensively about for its ability to improve cardiac function, help with congestive heart failure, and prevent heart attacks and strokes. When I read

Ling's work, everything started coming together. G-strophan-thin (ouabain) does not work on the sodium-potassium pump. Rather, it is one of the primary catalysts, if not *the* primary cata-lyst, for the phase changes within our cells, particularly the cells of the heart. Once g-strophanthin is bound, even at almost infinitesimally small doses, changes occur within the cell that exclude sodium and concentrate potassium and reenergize the entirety of the cell. G-strophanthin, made in our adrenal glands and supported by an extract of the seeds made from the *Strophanthus gratus* plant, is, as I suspected, the Gerson diet in pill or drop form.

While there is much to be done to understand how to use *Strophanthus* seed extracts with cancer patients, there are a num-ber of studies that already demonstrate its usefulness.[6] Still, the problem of its less-than-dramatic effectiveness clearly means that stimulating the sodium-potassium pump is not the whole story. There are other components of this system that need exploration and understanding.

CHAPTER SEVEN

Plant and Mushroom Medicines

I n all of my lectures, in all of my books, including this book, I discuss not only the subject at hand, in this case cancer, but also a way of seeing the world. While I can make no claims that my way of seeing the world is somehow better than the "usual" way, I do think that the underlying approach I am advocating belongs in the conversation about how human beings can and should attempt to understand complex subjects. My approach, which is also certainly not unique to me, is more synthetic than analytic, more expansive than reductionist, and relies more on the capacities of the individual than on the dictates of an authority or authoritative group. A few examples may help explain what I mean here.

In the early days of my practice I would do regular calls with some of my similar-aged anthroposophical medical colleagues to go over cases and develop treatment strategies for different people and different conditions. We all had different approaches to medicine based on our varied backgrounds, knowledge bases, and interests, so our process together also served as a way to hear different perspectives. One of my colleagues was interested in data-based information about his patients as an aid in guiding therapy. One way he did this was to run mineral analyses of the blood, hair, and urine of many of his patients. He took this information and, using different formulas, figured out which mineral supplements to give his patients, raising levels that were too low and bringing down levels that were too high. His hope was that over time, as the mineral levels normalized, the patient's condition would improve.

One time, after compiling all this data, he showed me the numbers and the subsequent formula that he had devised that would accomplish this normalization. I looked at it and said it looked familiar. I went and got my jar of Celtic sea salt, the only salt I have used in my food for decades. Celtic sea salt is one of the few commercially available salts that simply slowly evaporates the water from ocean water, leaving all the minerals present in the salt intact. This is in sharp contrast to normal commercial table salt, which is typically only sodium chloride (NaCl). To my surprise, I discovered that my friend's complex formula to rebalance his patient's mineral levels was almost identical to the composition of Celtic sea salt.

I am not criticizing this more analytical approach per se, but I am pointing out that often one can arrive at the same conclusion without the analytical, reductionist steps. In other words, as was pointed out in chapter 4, the mineral composition of human blood is identical to that found in the sea. Every human being, in their quest to maintain or improve their health, should strictly avoid all processed or unbalanced salt or mineral preparations. If you are too low in calcium, for example, and you supplement it, this will impact the amount of phosphorus in your blood (which will impact the tissues and cells). So then you supplement phosphorus, but this affects the amount of silica in your blood, which then affects your iron and so on. Once, when I went down this frustrating and futile path, I threw up my hands and just said, "The heck with this. I'll just eat Celtic salt and will probably be fine." I sometimes refer to this path as the medicine of complexity, meaning the human being and life itself are so complex as to be basically unknowable. Faced with this complexity, I use an approach that involves trying to find some basic truths that can guide us. One of these truths is that humans need to be exposed to all the minerals that exist in rough proportions to those found in our blood or in the sea. There are strong scientific reasons for this, reasons that emerge if one commits to big-picture synthetic thinking.

In the 1980s I was exposed to the work of Louis Kervran on the subject of biological transmutations.[1] We are taught in science class that the elements of the periodic table are inviolable basic units. In other words, calcium is always calcium; it is neither created anew nor changes into zinc, iron, or any other element. This is an axiomatic principle in science. What Kervran pointed out is that if you examine a closed system in nature such as a bird egg, you will see that the elements that make up a newly laid egg are different from the elements that make up the newly hatched chick. An egg is a perfect system to study because there is no possibility of any elements being somehow added to the egg during the course of its maturation; it is completely closed, with no interaction with the outside world. The curious thing about this example is that even though the scientific stance on it is that the change that occurs is impossible, it is also obvious that something profound has happened in changing an egg yolk into a chick. It is not surprising, therefore, that the chick is made out of different elements than the yolk (and white, or albumen).

The process is not simply a matter of rearranging the elements to change the egg contents into a chick; it is a more profound transformation than that. This, I submit, is obvious to anyone until they have it "scienced" out of them.

Kervran even went further and spelled out in detail the usual types of transformations that take place in nature. For example, it appears it is easy for living systems to transform silica into calcium. This explains the enthusiasm laying chickens have for eating silica chips, called mica, which contain no calcium, but which farmers know produce thick, healthy eggshells. For science this makes no sense. For someone who lets the phenomenon speak without prejudice, the transformation is simple and easy to understand.

When confronted with examples like this, most scientists say the energy required to accomplish these types of transmutations would need to be more powerful than the most powerful nuclear reactors and, while nuclear reactors do, in fact, create the energy that can accomplish some of these mineral transformations, that amount of energy is not possible within a tiny chick or egg. Yes; except it's a fact, it happens, and it's obvious it happens. This can only mean that the life energy of any living being is, in fact, more powerful than any nuclear reactor ever devised. (And when I say *power* I don't mean destructive capacity—I mean creative capacity. While we know how to build energy systems and devices that destroy, we unfortunately have no clue how to create systems that sustain and support life.)

The point I'm trying to make is that there are at least two principal ways of knowing. The first is the analytical, reductionist, mechanistic way of science. The second is a more synthetic, intuitive, observational approach. Not only do we need both, but the second approach is actually more effective when it comes to working with living systems and when it comes to healing, in particular. When the two are in conflict, as they so often are these days, the default approach should be to trust your observations and instincts.

There is an increasing disconnect between what we are told and, in particular, what we are told to think, compared to facts we observe in our own life. We need to learn to stop trusting experts, especially when their conclusions contradict our own experience. We see this phenomenon over and over in cancer medicine. So often people say their loved one was doing fine, they were convinced to do conventional cancer therapies, and soon after, their love one was dead. Believe what you see with your own eyes, and trust your heart to guide you in the right direction.

With that introduction, let's turn to some plant and mushroom medicines that have historically been used to treat cancer, something I have been involved with for over thirty years and with many hundreds of patients. The goal of this section will be to examine the primary plants and mushrooms that I (and many others) have used to help cancer patients over many decades. Most treatises on cancer and plant and mushroom medicines assume the usual causes of cancer are nucleus/DNA-based and then attempt to understand the basis for the benefits of these plants and mushrooms from that perspective. In other words, they use a reductionist, chemical, research-based approach to the study of these medicines. As I just outlined, my approach is different. I always start with a bigger picture, where I go from a wide perspective of the understanding of the disease and then move to an examination of the life of the plant to see how these two interact. It's not that I am opposed to adding the reductionist approach to our understanding, but if you start there, you often end up not being able to see the forest for the trees. We want to always start by asking the question: What does the plant or mushroom have to say to the human being? This question is, after all, the one that led people to discover plants and mushrooms as agents of healing in the first place.

Chaga

The first principle in this macroscopic approach to understanding healing plants and mushrooms is to understand what has historically been called the doctrine of signatures. This doctrine suggests we understand the therapeutic function of a plant or mushroom by comparing its features to the disease in question. Cancer, whatever its underlying causes, appears as a growth on or in the body of the person affected. It is an irregular, chaotic, disorganized sort of growth that is typically denser and more mineral-like than the surrounding tissue. Some cancerous growths—in particular the deadly skin cancer melanoma—are black masses of disorganized cells. All of these features of melanoma describe the normal growth habit of the parasitic polyporous fungus called chaga mushroom, or *Inonotus obliquus*.

As I describe various healing plants and mushrooms for cancer, the theme of parasitic growth will often emerge; it's the growth habit of most solid tumors. Chaga, used for millennia as a cancer medicine in Siberia and other northern locations, grows like a black, chaotic, dense mass to the point of being almost mineral-like. It is a fungus growing almost exclusively on the birch trees of the northern forests. It derives its nutrition from "sucking" the sap of the trees, much like cancer derives its nutrition from "stealing" it from the blood of the patient. Yet chaga doesn't kill the tree, unlike cancer, but eventually comes to a stable and even harmonious relationship with the tree—this relationship is significant for understanding its therapeutic potential. Some who study chaga have suggested that birch trees that harbor chaga may have some inherent advantage compared to those that don't. In other words, we could say that chaga shows us the way to healing through coexistence, even with what could be a deadly parasite. The lesson is: Be careful who or what you kill. This is a lesson we've also dramatically learned through the use of antibiotics that kill our beneficial gut flora in the misguided quest to rid our bodies of infections.

I first heard about the use of chaga for cancer as a teenager, when I was an avid reader of Russian novels. Aleksandr Solzhenitsyn's *Cancer Ward*, supposedly an autobiographical novel, was his description of the horrors of a Siberian cancer ward for political prisoners. When the main character developed a deadly cancer (probably a melanoma), he ran away into the forest rather than submitting himself to the horrors of "treatment" in the cancer ward. In the forest, he was given a tea made from a fungus growing on birch trees (it could only have been chaga), which cured him of cancer and eventually led to his escape from the

Gulag. That dramatic depiction of chaga's healing powers stuck with me and resurfaced years later when I read that Rudolf Steiner thought that birch trees have a strong affinity for skin ailments, including skin cancer. Knowing the remarkable similarity of growth habit and appearance of chaga to melanoma, I consulted the medical literature and found that birch trees synthesize a protein called betulin, which exhibits protective activity against many types of cancer cells, melanoma in particular.[2] I was not surprised to find that chaga collects this betulin from the birch sap and concentrates it in its fruiting body, the part used to make chaga tea.[3] Chaga is a dramatic case in which the synthetic approach to understanding a plant or mushroom as a medicine aligns perfectly with a reductionist approach.

As Goethe taught, we must learn to read the book of nature, and in this way the plant or mushroom will demonstrate paths to healing for anyone who has the openness to see. We must see the overall picture, the statement it makes to the world. It is telling us about its place in nature and its relation to the human being. The chaga is essentially saying, "I am the way to restore balance and harmony when black growths emerge from your skin and threaten to overwhelm your life. I can help you come back to this harmonious relationship that I myself have found with my friend the birch trees." Then you can use reductionist science to confirm your understanding. With chaga, the two approaches line up perfectly.

The next step is to give the medicine and observe what happens. For example, I had a patient in a dangerous situation with melanoma who used chaga as a tea and alcoholic extract, each of which concentrates different chemicals and elements from the fungus. My patient was in her mid-sixties when she had a recurrence of a malignant melanoma that was originally found and excised three years earlier. With melanomas, recurrence is often an ominous sign and a development associated with a poor prognosis. Since there are few conventional medical treatments that work for people with malignant melanoma, she sought me out for alternative care. Five years later, to the surprise of her conventional oncologists and a melanoma specialist, she is free of disease and claims to be in better health now than she was five years ago. The only glitch during those five years was a small spot that showed up in a brain scan that quickly resolved with the addition of silver acupuncture needles. Otherwise, the backbone of her therapy was a change in diet along the lines I describe in chapter 12, a few years of mistletoe therapy, and lots of chaga tea and chaga tincture.

This is just one story, and taking chaga is just one of many changes this patient made in her life, but over the years, many of my melanoma patients have seemingly defied the unfavorable odds and lived long and healthy lives with the simple addition of a good diet and chaga mushroom. (In my estimation, chaga can be considered almost a specific therapy for melanoma.) And in every good outcome I have ever seen with melanoma, and many of the good outcomes I've seen with various types of cancer, the common response patients give years later is: "I stuck to the diet." Or "I never missed a mistletoe injection." Or "I drank chaga tea or took chaga drops every day." I am not suggesting these cases provide proof of chaga's efficacy, but after billions of dollars and fifty years of effort that have achieved little or no progress, can't we agree that it's time to at least examine this new approach, both in our understanding of how to conceptualize illness and in the actual medicines we use? Chaga needs to be part of the conversation.

Burdock

One plant in the quest to understand and treat cancer is the humble burdock, also known as *Arctium lappa*. As one of the founders of my family's vegetable and spice powder business, Dr. Cowan's Garden, I am also the head gardener. Because our Napa garden is located in prime wine country, on an organic vineyard, it is important for me to understand the nature of each plant in our garden. In particular, we are cautious about introducing invasive species. This is why, even though I love to eat burdock and we have an organically grown burdock powder in our line of products, I will never plant burdock in our garden. I am grateful there are people who have healthy, organic burdock gardens from whom we can source our product, because this otherwise nondescript, unremarkable plant does have one remarkable characteristic: an ability to invade and overtake everything in its path. As anyone who spends time in the woods will know, burdock produces burrs that put Velcro to shame in their ability to attach to and embed in whatever they touch. Burdock's burrs end up on your clothes, attached to your skin, and in your dog's fur. And once you have one burdock plant in your garden or on your property, no matter what you do, you will never eradicate it. It will propagate itself through seeds on the burrs that animals will carry to far-flung areas of your property. Tenacity and invasiveness, those are the encapsulation of the qualities of burdock.

Is it any wonder, then, that when confronted with cancer, a disease whose danger comes from its tenacity, invasiveness, and near impossibility of eradication, we see the humble burdock root as a predominant ingredient in all the famous herbal remedies, on virtually all continents? It is as if the plants paint a mosaic of the different qualities of whatever disease they can help address. Cancer is the most tenacious, aggressive disease humans will ever confront. Once it lands in a person, an ongoing battle to eradicate it ensues. This tenacity is the nature of burdock. This sort of synthetic thinking not only helps us understand the disease, but clears a therapeutic path for us to follow.

It is worthwhile to check our synthetic understanding of burdock with the reductionist approach. Numerous studies confirm the therapeutic potential of burdock root, which contains a lignan compound called arctigenin, for cancer patients. A recent study confirms that burdock root's therapeutic potential is based on its ability to deprive the tumors of the glucose they need to fuel their growth.[4] Another study shows the combined effect of green tea, curcumin, and burdock root on breast cancer cells.[5] And, finally, a 2018 review summarizes decades of studies showing the therapeutic potential of burdock root on a number of different types of cancer, including stomach, lung, liver, and colon cancer, thanks to the arctigenin in it.[6] Changing how we think unlocks healing avenues that would otherwise keep us locked in a dead end of details and therapeutic failure.

Turmeric

These days most people have heard about the therapeutic potential of turmeric (*Curcuma longa*) root and its active ingredient, the polyphenol curcumin, in the treatment of a variety of diseases. There are cases, reports, and studies showing turmeric/curcumin to be an effective treatment for arthritis, neurodegenerative diseases such as Alzheimer's, and chronic inflammation. At last count there are 4,660 PubMed references to curcumin and cancer. While not all studies show dramatically positive effects, there is no doubt at this point that turmeric/curcumin is a potent medicine for many conditions, including cancer. The search now is for the strategy to make it as effective and bioavailable to patients as possible.

I was first exposed to turmeric/curcumin as a medicine in the early 1980s. In studying anthroposophical medicine, I learned about a group of medicines called the dorons, which were formulas given by Rudolf Steiner directly to the working group of doctors he trained. Each doron was specific to an organ, function, or disease, and the word *doron* apparently translated roughly as "gift to." So, *cardiodoron* was the gift to the heart, *renodoron* was the gift to the kidney, and so on. Steiner not only detailed the composition of the dorons, he also gave specific instructions as to how the medicine was to be made. In each case, the pharmaceutical preparation was different and was based on some principle that was relevant to the given organ.

Cardiodoron, for example, was made under certain temperature conditions due to Steiner's understanding of the connection between the heart and warmth. One of the most important dorons was choleodoron, or gift to the bile (or gall bladder). The composition of choleodoron is the roots of two plants well known to traditional and herbal medicine: turmeric and greater celandine. Interestingly, both of these plant medicines are currently being studied for their anticancer effects.

The gall bladder and bile ducts together function as an outflow tube for the passage of bile from the liver to the small intestine. The analogy that best describes this is that the primary function of the liver is to bag the body's garbage (the waste products) to be taken out to curb by the flow of the bile. The liver uses its various enzymes and conjugation pathways to make waste soluble through conversions performed by its enzymes, then dissolve these now-soluble toxins in the bile. The bile then flows outward from the liver into the duodenum, where the dissolved toxins can be mixed with the stool and expelled from the body.

If either of these steps, sometimes called phase 1 and phase 2 of liver detoxification, is impaired, sickness can result. If the liver enzymes are ineffective, weak, absent, or somehow poorly functioning, a person is not able to convert the many toxins humans are exposed to into their soluble form. If this conversion doesn't happen, the toxins can't be easily excreted and many problems result. Or, if the liver is functioning properly but the bile flow is weak, the body may overfill with soluble toxins, much like a house in which nobody takes the garbage out to the curb. In this case, as well, serious disease can result.

For as long as there has been herbal medicine, there have been plant medicines that were used for their choleretic (bile stimulation) effect. Almost all of them, not coincidentally, have bitter, yellow-colored "sap" in their roots. Three of the most common examples of these are turmeric, greater celandine, and the well-known herb for treating infections—goldenseal. One could say the signature of all choleretic plants is that they concentrate bilelike, bitter, yellow substances in their root. When ingested, these bitter substances stimulate bile flow, an effect that is similar to the ending of the garbage collection strikes that many times threatened to bring cities like New York to their knees. The bile can flow, the body can rid itself of poisons, and the liver is once more free to do its job. Without a robust bile flow, we become a toxic soup, at first prone to infection (stagnant bile is known to be a common breeding place for pathogen growth), later prone to the toxic condition we call cancer. It is for this reason that coffee enemas and numerous other detoxification maneuvers are part of every holistic cancer program. Coffee given as an enema directly dilates the common bile duct, and this is arguably the strongest, most direct approach to improving bile flow. For me, this is the primary reason turmeric/ curcumin is a dramatically potent cancer medicine. I am not denying that curcumin has direct effects on the growth and properties of cancer cells, but for turmeric to take its rightful place as a cancer therapy, we should not lose sight of the plant itself, which loudly informs us that "I am a plant that through my yellow bitterness stimulates bile flow and your ability to keep yourself free of unwanted garbage."

There is some interesting evidence that in times past herbal medicines were more effective than they are today. While there could be many reasons for this, there are three possibilities that I think are especially relevant. First, in my reading of traditional medicine tomes or about the lifestyles of traditional people, together with my two years of living in rural, traditional Africa, it became clear that herbs had a much different place in the lives of traditional people than they do for modern Americans. People native to India, in the rural areas, generally ate between two and six tablespoons per day of turmeric, always dissolved in ghee and mixed with black pepper. Modern research has shown that we need to take curcumin with fat in order for our bodies to absorb it and that mixing turmeric with black pepper also facilitates absorption. There is a big difference between eating turmeric as a part of one's daily diet and taking it as a pill, no matter how sophisticated the delivery system. I am not denying that curcumin, properly delivered, might be an effective and safer chemo "drug" than the ones we use today, but I think we should not discount the fact that the main therapeutic effect of turmeric is the stimulation of the bile and that can only come about as a result of actually tasting, eating the turmeric.

The second reason herbs are less effective today is our gut flora is imbalanced. When we ingest herbs, our gut microbes need to convert them into secondary metabolites in order for our bodies to make use of them. If our gut flora is imbalanced, as is the case for virtually all modern people, this conversion doesn't occur. For this reason, whenever we use plant medicines, we should do so in combination with a gut-restoration program.

Finally, a lot of herbs are ineffective because people grow the wrong species, they grow them in places that are unsuitable for the concentration of the plant's active components, or the growing techniques themselves produce unhealthy, even toxic, plants. There is no effective herb for cancer or for any other ailment that has been grown in soil treated with glyphosate (Roundup), since glyphosate inhibits the formation of the secondary metabolites of the plants that are the active ingredients in disease prevention. If we want to optimize our therapy, and we always do with cancer treatment, we need to procure the finest herbs traditionally grown in the location that best suits them. We need cardamom from the cloud forest in Guatemala, nutmeg from the Zanzibar islands off of Tanzania, and turmeric from biodynamic farms in either India or the Hawaiian islands. You can taste, smell, and feel the difference. Herbs grown in their homes can express their true potential. If you are coping with serious diseases, it is essential to ingest plants that are expressing their full potency. Only then do the plants become true healers. Later, in chapter 12, I offer suggestions on how to implement the use of turmeric in your own healing program.

Ashitaba

Ashitaba, otherwise known as *Angelica keiskei*, is a plant that is fairly new to me. It is the only edible member of the *Angelica* family of plants, the most famous example of which is *Angelica archangelica*. This auspicious name, meaning the gift of the arch-angels to the angels, was reportedly hung in every doorway in medieval Europe as the only effective way to ward off the plague. Ashitaba is native to the Pacific Rim, and is mostly grown and used in rich volcanic soils in Japan, the Philippines, and Indonesia. Ashitaba has a few remarkable characteristics that make it worth exploring.

First, ashitaba is one of the most nutritious vegetables you can eat. Containing more nutrients per gram than such super-vegetables as kale, and rich in soluble vitamins and minerals, ashitaba is worth including in your diet simply as a source of vitamins, minerals, and phytonutrients. But the real magic of the ashitaba plant comes in its thick, sticky yellow sap that oozes out of the cut stem.

One of our family's primary reasons for founding Dr. Cowan's Garden was to try and make ashitaba available to American consumers. There are a few ashitaba teas or powders available on the internet, but none is truly organically grown, and none of them have the taste, smell, or feel of true ashitaba. As the head gardener, I had to learn how to grow enough ashitaba plants in our Napa garden to meet our growing demand. This, in spite of hearing from an Asian grower that we will never get ashitaba to grow in California.

During my three-year battle with ashitaba, I have learned a lot about the plant and why it may become a major player in the world of cancer therapeutics. First, ashitaba has strong life and growth forces, perhaps the reason why its common name is *tomorrow's leaf*. This name arose because if you cut a leaf today, tomorrow there will be a new one in its place. This strong force of growth, which unchecked is similar to the uncontrolled growth we call cancer, is seemingly held in check by a kind of natural chemo chemical in the plant's stem, called chalcone. Chalcones are in the family of aromatic ketones, fatty substances associated with ketone bodies, which I cover in chapter 8, on the ketogenic diet. These chalcones are powerful antioxidants and are currently being intensely investigated for their ability to stop a variety of cancer growths. An excerpt from a review article about the potential for ashitaba chalcones in oncology stated: "Based on the current studies, chalcones are highly multifunctional and their targets cover almost all of the actions of tumor cells, including growth, proliferation, invasion and metastasis."[7]

In other words, many aspects of cancer cells—their ability to grow, proliferate, spread, and invade other tissues—are addressed by ashitaba's chalcones. Just like a few decades ago when it was discovered that yew trees contained chemicals called taxanes that would stop cancerous growth, it is possible that one of the next big discoveries will be the potential of ashitaba chalcones. My theory is that we would have more success and safety if, instead of continually focusing on a single chemical made by the plant, we worked with the entirety of the plant.

Ashitaba requires great care to grow. I learned that any mistake—too much heat, not enough water, gopher infestations, you name it—and the ashitaba plant will become weak and the sap will be either scant or thin. Occasionally, we got it right and were rewarded with highly aromatic, thick, sticky yellow sap, rich in ashitaba chalcones. It is this healthy plant that has the healing potential, potential that will take great skill and patience to unlock. In appendix A I'll share where to buy and how to use ashitaba powder and chalcones.

Mistletoe

Our final plant is the undisputed king of natural cancer medicines: mistletoe. No other natural medicine has such a long history of usage (over a hundred years), clinical trials, and basic

research as does mistletoe. Clinical usage and research unequivo-
cally demonstrate that mistletoe use for cancer is safe,[8] extends
quality of life when used in clinical trials with cancer patients,[9]
successfully treats pleural effusions that result from lung cancer,[10]
improves survival in patients with stage 4 lung cancer,[11] and
improves survival in patients with stage 4 cancer of the pancreas.[12]
In addition, in some cases mistletoe use can result in remissions,
such as remission in a patient with non-Hodgkin's lymphoma[13]
or a patient cured of cancer that had metastasized to his skull.[14]
Installation of mistletoe extracts in the bladder of patients with
bladder cancer has been associated with improved outcomes and
occasionally full remission.[15] And scores of published papers
document the mechanism by which mistletoe extracts have a
positive effect on all markers and parameters associated with the
cancer process, including one in particular comparing the mechanism of action of mistletoe extracts with that of Coley's toxins.[16]
Without a doubt, mistletoe extracts should be considered settled
science in the annals of therapeutic interventions that improve
the outcome for patients with cancer. The questions that I wish
to address are: What is mistletoe? How does it work? And how
does it fit in with my central thesis that cancer is fundamentally a
problem of the cytoplasmic water?

In more than thirty-five years as a practicing physician, I
have treated almost all of my cancer patients, numbering in the
hundreds, with some form of mistletoe. This has given me a lot
of experience with how to use mistletoe and what we can expect
from it. Experience has taught me that while I still consider
mistletoe therapy the backbone of any holistic cancer treatment,
it's not perfect. I also hope to make clear the reasons mistletoe
cannot be the end of the line in cancer treatment but rather is a
useful step along the path.

Generally, my experience with mistletoe is that patients who,
usually as a result of surgery, have no active disease (on scans)
will have a very favorable outcome as a result of mistletoe use.
The melanoma patient I described earlier in this chapter who

used chaga mushroom to such positive effect is alive, well, and free of disease four years following her recurrence. This is an extremely unusual outcome for melanoma patients, and the outcome is probably also due to her use of mistletoe.

Another patient originally consulted me about her situation with osteoporosis and back pain that developed following her conventional treatment for an aggressive fallopian tube cancer. After a recurrence of the cancer in her lymph nodes and pelvis, she was treated with radiation and ended up with a lot of back pain and spinal fractures. As she described it: "Several fractures in my spine led me to my finding Dr. Thomas Cowan. Through natural substances he healed my bones in a matter of weeks. He asked me what I was doing about my cancer. I replied, 'Nothing. I hope it is gone.'"

Generally, this is a situation where the cancer would usually return, so to be proactive I suggested she start mistletoe therapy. She was fine for years until, as is often the case, her physician husband had his own health crisis. The stress in her life, along with stopping the mistletoe therapy during a hectic time, coincided with a return of cancer in her lung. At the time, a surgical debulking procedure was performed and she was told her prognosis was poor. In spite of this, she refused chemotherapy and restarted mistletoe. Now, almost two years since that procedure, she continues on her mistletoe therapy and is alive and well. Her friends and doctors refer to her as a miracle patient because, in spite of her poor prognosis, she seems to be flourishing and living an active, disease-free life.

The principle is simple: If you are able to remove the original tumor, mistletoe therapy can be a safe, effective, and easy-to-administer long-term follow-up strategy. A prominent surgeon was diagnosed with a malignant cancer of the kidney. He had a successful surgery that obtained clear margins, but unfortunately a follow-up PET scan showed increased activity in a lymph node next to the aorta. This lymph activity is often a sign of a poor prognosis, and his consultation with an oncologist was not reassuring. He was told he had three to five years to live whether or not he underwent chemotherapy, as chemotherapy is known to not work well for this particular type of cancer.

This patient, however, had many years of contact with physicians based in Germany and to his surprise many of his physician friends urged him to eschew chemotherapy and try mistletoe therapy instead. He contacted me, we started mistletoe therapy, and he has used it as a stand-alone therapy ever since. At his five-year diagnosis "anniversary," a follow-up PET scan revealed that he is free of disease. As of this writing he is alive, well, fully active in his life, and grateful for the choice he made five years ago.

Occasionally, there are cases with very poor prognoses after surgical removal of a tumor but in which long-lasting, almost miraculous recoveries occur. I had an acquaintance who was the young mother of four children when she was found to have stage 4 colon cancer with a large metastasis to her liver, a diagnosis that carries an extremely poor prognosis. She was treated by a friend of mine with the support of an oncologist at Johns Hopkins who realized that conventional chemotherapy had little to offer her. The amazing sequel to this story is that now, ten years free of any disease, almost unheard of in this situation, she is spearheading the first clinical trial of mistletoe therapy in the United States. Here is her story:

> *Every day I am filled with such gratefulness for the gift of healing I received in overcoming stage-4 colon cancer that statistically gave me a less than 8% chance of surviving. I attribute a large part of my healing to mistletoe. I was the very same age and had the very same type of cancer that took my father's life, my grandmother's life, and half of her siblings as well. Discovering that the survivorship of stage 4 colon cancer with metastasis to the liver was less than 8%, my husband, Jimmy, and I made the decision to forgo chemotherapy and radiation, as it would not have increased my chances of survival. On the conventional side,*

I had incredible surgeons who removed the cancer from my colon and liver, and I had a great oncologist who was willing to monitor me with scans and blood work even though I was not going to follow his standard protocol of chemotherapy and radiation. I wish there were more oncologists and physicians . . . who are humble enough to work with their patients when considering a patient's desire for a more complementary or holistic approach. On the complementary side, [my doctor] changed my internal environment to fight any remaining cancer after surgeries with a plant based diet, homeopathy, cancer fighting supplements, and Mistletoe injections. I had faced, fought and overcome cancer.

What is mistletoe's story and how does it work to help cancer patients? Well, we all know the story of mistletoe's connection to Christmas. The birth of Jesus is a story of light breaking through at the darkest time, a story of hope and overcoming our toughest challenges. Mistletoe, unlike most "normal" plants, is present in the Christmas story because it has liberated itself from the usual flower-in-the-spring, fruit-in-the-summer rhythm to hold off the ripening of its berries until around the time of the winter solstice, the darkest time of year. Mistletoe is a semiparasitic plant, getting its nutrients from the sap of the trees it parasitizes. It grows in a circular form, much like a tumor growing on our internal organs, equally in all directions. Mistletoe is undifferentiated; all parts of the plant—root, leaves, flower, stem—are morphologically about the same, which is again reminiscent of the undifferentiated primitive growth habit of the typical cancer mass. If you look at a tree "infected" with mistletoe, it looks like a tree with multiple tumors; as with chaga and its host the birch tree, until very late in the infection, trees with mistletoe seem to thrive. Mistletoe is the picture in nature of the coexistence of undifferentiated growth with its host. It reminds us that this is not, as Nixon proposed, a war on cancer, but is a journey of coexistence. It seems that until we learn that vital concept, we are destined to promote a warlike consciousness and to have cancer be a major player in our culture. Mistletoe demonstrates the way out of this primitive and destructive mind-set, a mind-set that forms the foundation of our modern approach to oncology. We want to kill everything that is not us. In attempting to do so, we destroy ourselves.

When Rudolf Steiner, the first person we know of to propose mistletoe as a medicine for cancer, was asked "What does mistletoe do?" he gave two answers. The first was that mistletoe simulates a bacterial infection. The second was that mistletoe is *the* medicine to heal the etheric body. The first of these responses makes me wonder if Steiner, who was not a medical person at all, was aware of work going on at that time with Coley's toxins and other attempts to treat cancer by provoking febrile responses in patients. Coley was developing ways to avoid giving his cancer patients infections like erysipelas and pneumonia and instead simulate the fevers that accompany these infections with toxins derived from different bacteria. The infection is not the therapy; the body's fight to overcome the infection is the therapy. Specifically, fever with its inherent stimulation of the innate or cell-mediated immune response from an immunological point of view has been one of cancer's greatest healers for centuries. Mistletoe therapy, given at the correct dose in the proper manner, can and does stimulate this fever response in sick patients. This has been and will always be a main therapeutic approach to the problem of cancer.

From the perspective of the cytoplasmic water and cancer connection that is the basis of this book, I attribute the power of fever, or hyperthermia, or saunas, or any warmth therapy to its ability to heal cytoplasmic gels that for whatever reason have become poisoned, distorted, and dysfunctional. As a result of this distortion they can no longer generate the energy needed to run the life of the cell; they are no longer able to create the separation of charge from the inside to the outside of the cell; the cell loses its energy, clumps together, and undergoes transformation into a cancerous growth. Anything one can do to heat the gel and allow it to cleanse itself through fever in order to reconstitute a more healthy cytoplasm is in the direction of healing. Mistletoe, through its stimulation of warmth in the human organism, helps toward this end.

Steiner's *etheric body*, the fluid or water part of the human organism, was also referred to as the *formative force* or the *life force* of the organism. The etheric body is exactly what is missing in that heap of chemicals that comes from a carrot (chapter 3). The carrot is a combination of these chemicals, along with a formative, water-based body or force that imbues it with life. According to Steiner, when this life, this water body, is ill at its extreme, that is what we call cancer. Mistletoe, he said, is the medicine that can begin to heal this etheric body of the ill patient. (That, in a nutshell, is the point of this book.)

When we combine these two perspectives—the more metaphorical understanding of Steiner and the research showing mistletoe extract as an immune stimulation, cytotoxic (kills cancer cells), apoptosis-promoting medicine—we can see that mistletoe is well placed to take its rightful role as a centerpiece of any true cancer therapy. However, mistletoe is also a gentle medicine, which means that it is often not enough.

To some extent this is due to the tentativeness of modern doctors to stimulate high fevers in their patients. We can do this with mistletoe injections, particularly given intravenously, but it is a dramatic therapy that not all doctors are willing to prescribe and not all patients are willing to undergo. The lack of effectiveness of mistletoe could also be due in part to the preparations themselves. There are currently about six brands of mistletoe available worldwide. Each has its proponents and detractors; none is as immunologically active as I would hope. In chapter 12, I give precise instructions on how to use mistletoe injections, including the type of mistletoe that I have found most successful. And, finally, while mistletoe is undoubtedly a medicine for the etheric or water body, I propose that in conjunction with its use we also need to examine the nature of the water itself in the cell. In other words, we can stimulate or encourage all we want, but at some point we need to look directly at the intracellular water as well as attempt to understand and harness this actual etheric force to which mistletoe is pointing us. It is to these important areas that we turn our attention next.

CHAPTER EIGHT

The Ketogenic Diet

A few months ago I was listening to an episode of the *Joe Rogan Show* about whether a vegan diet or Paleo diet is better for preventing or managing heart disease. I happened to know both of the guests, each a respected leader in his field of expertise. The vegan cardiologist gave an eloquent explanation about how there was virtually no heart disease in this country during the early part of the twentieth century. Then things began to change around the Second World War, until heart disease escalated to near epidemic proportions. In my opinion, the debate should have ended at that point with a simple question: "As you pointed out, there was virtually no heart disease in the early part of the twentieth century. How many people ate a vegan diet at that time?" The answer, of course is zero. How can anyone claim that by eliminating those foods such as cream, butter, and eggs that were considered "health foods" at a time when people had no heart disease, we would somehow eliminate heart disease? It defies logic.

Something similar has happened with the diet and cancer connection. Cancer was rare in the early twentieth century. Family doctors went their whole careers without seeing a single case of breast cancer. Today most people know someone in their immediate neighborhood, if not their own family, with breast cancer, a disease now affecting people at younger and younger ages. All this has occurred during the past fifty years or so, since a vegetarian or vegan diet became the accepted holistic cancer diet. Never mind that people rarely got cancer when almost no one ate a vegan or vegetarian diet. Furthermore, numerous anthropology studies and books have confirmed the absence of cancer in indigenous people even though none ate a vegetarian or vegan diet.[1] The tide has started to turn recently and people seem much more open to exploring different diets for cancer, especially since the publication of Dr. Thomas Seyfried's *Cancer as a Metabolic Disease*.

As we saw in chapter 2, Seyfried posited that the fundamental defect in cancer is dysfunction of the mitochondria. The mitochondria are essentially primitive bacteria, complete with their own genome, that reside in the cytoplasm of most mammalian cells. The role of the mitochondria is to produce ATP, the so-called energy molecule of the body. In return for being their internal power plants, the cells supply the mitochondria with nutrients, antioxidants in particular, which allow the mitochondria to function smoothly and efficiently.

The Warburg effect, also discussed in chapter 2, is that all cancer cells have defects in their mitochondrial function that prevent these mitochondria from producing the energy needed for optimal cellular function. These defects can be genetic in nature, or from radiation, coal tar, and an endless list of other carcinogens. As a result, the cells shift to the glycolytic pathway and start to produce energy through glycolysis, otherwise known as fermentation. This is a primitive, inefficient way to produce ATP, one used by single-celled organisms and fungi. The consequence of this glycolytic shift is that the cells, like primitive organisms, get stuck in a continual growth cycle. They lose connection to the tissue they are embedded in and essentially behave like any single-celled organism, which attempts to continually grow and divide as long as there is an adequate source of food. This primitive pattern becomes the growth that is the hallmark of the cancer process.

As I discussed in chapter 2, the modern proof that this glycolytic shift does, in fact, occur with virtually all cancer cells is that PET scans, the most sophisticated technique of modern oncology for detecting cancer cells and cancer growth patterns, take advantage of this change in energy production to detect cancer. Healthy cells, using their mitochondria to produce ATP, make thirty-six molecules of ATP from each molecule of glucose. Glycolysis, in contrast, is an incomplete process and therefore only produces two molecules of ATP for each molecule of glucose.

Therefore, a cell relying on glycolysis must have access to eighteen times the amount of glucose in order to survive. Cancer cells, in order to survive energetically, shift their metabolism to maximize glucose uptake. While they are rarely able to achieve eighteen times the glucose uptake as a normal cell, they can achieve between two and five times the uptake. This is identified by giving the patient radioactively labeled glucose.

If this radioactively labeled glucose is picked up by a collection of cells, then by definition those cells must be cancer cells. There are no other cells that have that type of glucose dysregulation. This picture then allows the radiologist to "see" the cancer and give an assessment of how active it is based on its glucose uptake. To dispute the centrality of this Warburg effect in cancer is to dispute the fundamental basis of modern oncology diagnostic practices.

As I have pointed out, placing the source of cancer in the mitochondria is consistent with my premise that cancer is a loss of cellular integrity due to deterioration of the intracellular gel structure. Furthermore, once we understand that the role of ATP in any mammalian organism is not as an energy source, but as the molecule that unfolds the cytoplasmic proteins and therefore structures the intracellular water into an effective gel, the whole picture begins to make sense. This intracellular water structuring is accomplished by the ATP attaching to the ends of the intracellular proteins. As a result of this attachment, the proteins unfold and are then able to function as the seed points for the intracellular water to form itself into a gel. The ATP in our cells plays the same role that heat plays in the formation of Jell-O. With Jell-O you mix proteins with water and then you heat the mixture, which unfolds the proteins. These unfolded proteins bond with water that upon cooling creates the gel we call Jell-O. Without sufficient ATP, because of damaged mitochondria and the ensuing glycolytic shift, the cell is no longer able to structure its intracellular gel. Since it is the intracellular gel that is responsible for the distribution of sodium and potassium across the cell membrane, this distribution will no longer be efficiently performed. The result is a cell without a charge that inevitably will clump together with the surrounding cells, forming itself into the characteristic tumor we see in cancer.

Second, the intracellular gel is the matrix in which cell division takes place. Without a properly structured matrix cell division, spindle formation, DNA transcription and translation, and all the other nuclear events we associate with cancer will become chaotic. These characteristic signs of cancer—abnormal number or types of chromosomes (aneuploidy), mutations, abnormal proteins synthesized—are all secondary effects of this primary mitochondrial/cytoplasmic defect. Only a blatantly superficial analysis would claim that aneuploidy or gene mutations are the primary event in cancer. This understanding is also consistent with the earlier analysis I cited in chapter 2, that transplanting a cancerous nucleus into a healthy cytoplasm does not produce a cancerous growth. Only when the cytoplasm is sick does cancer result.

The theory of the ketogenic diet follows directly from this understanding. That is, the normal cells can use either glucose (sugar) or fats as the substrate from which they synthesize ATP. Fats, and more specifically fatty acids, are the more efficient, generally preferred substrate for normal cells, but normal cells can and do use glucose to fuel the respiratory cycles in the mitochondria. Cancer cells, on the other hand, put all their eggs into the glucose basket. They are completely dependent on using glucose for fuel, having lost the ability to generate ATP from fatty acids. They will do everything possible to gain access to the needed glucose. First, they use the incoming glucose from the carbohydrates in food. Then, they use gluconeogenesis (new glucose formation) to produce the needed glucose from ingested protein. Then, as inevitably will happen, once these sources run out, they will facilitate the conversion of body fat into glucose to be used to produce ATP. Once the fat stores are exhausted, the cancer cells facilitate the conversion of the protein structure of the body into glucose to fuel the cancer growth. This explains the progression we see with cancer patients: At first, when the cancer cells are able to get the glucose they need from food, there is no weight loss, and usually there is only the feeling of fatigue. This stage reflects the shunting of the metabolism toward the cancer cells and therefore an ATP deficit for the normal cells and tissues. Next, the patient's fat is burned, associated with weight loss and worsening fatigue. In the final stage, the patient becomes cachectic as the structural proteins of the body are used as substrate for the cancer cells. This is the terminal stage, from which recovery is rare.

The theory behind the ketogenic diet for cancer essentially says that based on all of the above information, the logical conclusion is that if you stop eating all foods that contain carbohydrates, especially in the early phases, it will allow the normal cells to feed (on fats), and at the same time starve the cancer cells. Weakened cancer cells, deprived of their usual glucose diet and before they have started to break down the body's fat and protein stores, should allow a normally functioning immune system to clear out the cancer cells and restore the person to health.

During the past five years I have seen dozens of patients who have attempted systematic and rigorous ketogenic diets for their cancer. Most did exactly as outlined in the various books explaining the ketogenic approach to cancer: eating only twelve grams of carbohydrates per day, eating low protein, and calculating protein/fat ratios to keep them in the recommended range. Many people combined this with restricted total caloric intake as suggested by Seyfried; most inevitably lost weight as a result. In no case, however, did I see a reduction in their tumor burden or objective improvement in their overall condition. In other words, as is often the case in life, it seemed like a situation in which the theory simply didn't match up with the reality.

In trying to understand why this was so, I decided to run blood-sugar tests on people doing the ketogenic diet at various times and in a variety of situations. I ran fasting blood tests, blood tests after prolonged fasts (which puts one quickly into ketosis, or fat utilization mode), blood tests right after eating, and blood tests two, four, or five hours after eating. To my surprise, I never once saw a lower-than-expected blood sugar as a result of any of these dietary interventions. To be clear, for some, various fasting or ketogenic diets helped tremendously with elevated blood sugars and even diabetes. But, the important finding is that, as Seyfried suggests, in order to make a clinically relevant effect on the cancer cells through blood-sugar reduction, the sugar must drop in the low sixties or mid- to high fifties. In no case, no matter how little the patients ate, did their blood sugar drop at any time to less than seventy. The explanation for this can only be that the body has good reason and the hormonal mechanisms in place to prevent the blood sugar from dropping to these very low levels. Only under the most extreme situations, such as insulin-secreting tumors of the pancreas, will the body allow the blood sugar to drop to these therapeutically effective levels. For this reason, I fear the ketogenic diet approach, even the restricted-calorie ketogenic diet approach to cancer, is doomed to failure.

Seyfried and others are exploring possible drug approaches that work together with the ketogenic diet to lower the blood sugars to these more therapeutic levels, but as far as I know, they have found nothing even close to clinically useful at this point. At the same time as my direct experience tells me that the ketogenic dietary approach is not the solution to cancer, it also seems that there is something relevant and useful for cancer patients within it. For one thing, the typical high-quality ketogenic diet in many ways is similar to the general Nourishing Traditions type of diet I have advocated for decades; it's just lower in carbohydrates than most traditional diets. Additionally, an article came to my attention that may explain why a ketogenic approach, or what I would call a restricted-carbohydrate approach, still deserves attention and exploration. In a paper co-authored by Dominic D'Agostino, one of the premier ketogenic diet researchers in the world, research showed that animals who followed a ketogenic diet lowered the amount of deuterium in their cells and tissues.[2] Deuterium, as we will see, may actually be the missing link or mechanism for how a ketogenic diet might help cancer patients. It is the missing link between dietary therapy and the new science of water. It is to the role of deuterium and deuterium-depleted water in the cancer process that we next turn our attention.

CHAPTER NINE

Deuterium-Depleted Water

Not long ago, I had a meeting with the head of a cancer research lab to explore whether his lab had any interest in testing the role of deuterium-depleted water (DDW) to help understand the cause of and possible treatments for cancer. I presented him with the papers I will discuss below that show greater than twofold improvement in survival times for various classes of cancer patients, all peer-reviewed studies in conventional oncology journals, along with four published cases of patients with stage 4 lung cancer who achieved a durable remission solely through the use of DDW. He gave the papers a cursory look and asked what the mechanism is that explains how this water could possibly affect cancer patients. I gave a brief description of the new biology of water and its relevance for cancer. With a disgusted look, he said there were no reputable papers confirming this as a relevant factor in cancer, and said he was not interested in such a pursuit.

By the time I left, besides being glad to be done with the meeting, I was struck by how typical this is of the current science establishment. The overwhelming majority of published papers on cancer discuss it from the perspective of somatic mutations.

POTENTIAL THERAPIES

This is the accepted narrative and there is very little deviation from it. Therefore, if anyone presents a theory that is outside this framework, it is by definition unproven and unfounded and unworthy of anyone's time, money, or effort. The fact that the somatic mutation theory has led us nowhere and has been an almost total waste of money and resources is beside the point. What is even more shocking is that in spite of clear and convincing evidence that using DDW affects the prognosis of a person with cancer, this evidence is irrelevant to researchers in the current science establishment. Let's say I have no explanation for how and why DDW works. In a sane and just world shouldn't the *fact* that it does work prompt any honest scientist to say to herself, "I need to look differently at this problem so I understand how this is possible"? Instead, our science establishment, as personified by the researcher I met with, is more interested in promoting its own theories, no matter how tired, useless, or wasteful its approach. If you sense the contempt I feel as I write, you're correct. With so many people dying, and so much suffering, it's unconscionable to me that our science establishment is more concerned with careers and status quo than with urgently doing all we can to try to help people in desperate need.

Here is another example. The focus of this book, as you have undoubtedly gleaned by now, is to understand the new biology of water and how the "state" of our intracellular water affects our health. Up to now, I have mostly been describing this phenomenon and discussing various factors that influence our state of water. At some point, inevitably I had to turn my attention to the actual water itself that resides in our cells. Is water simply the "dead" H_2O molecule as science postulates or is water itself something much more? And if it is more, then is it possible that understanding water itself is the key to the kingdom of health and disease?

Asking the question in this way has led me to investigate the various waters of the earth, especially waters that are reputed to have healing properties. This inexorably led me to investigate

Lourdes, France, and its healing waters. The story goes that in 1858 an apparition claiming to be Mary visited a peasant girl named Bernadette, led her to a grotto where a spring appeared, and told her it contained waters with miraculous healing properties. After expressing the usual skepticism, confusion, and derision, villagers soon understood that something unusual and special was indeed happening at this grotto in Lourdes. In 1883, the Lourdes Medical Bureau, an independent commission consisting of doctors, pathologists, scientists, and others, was established to evaluate claims of unusual healing in order to validate them or reject them as the unproven stories of overly exuberant believers. The Catholic Church, which eventually canonized Bernadette, also established its own rules as to what constitutes a miraculous healing as a result of contact with the water at Lourdes.

From the study of the records of the Lourdes Medical Bureau and the findings of the Church council it is clear that the rules and procedures were actually quite rigorous. For example, for the international commission to certify that a medical healing has taken place, there must be documentation by medical authorities that the disease was present in the person before coming to Lourdes and an eyewitness account that the person was suffering from the disease. For example, if a person is paralyzed, they must present medical records stating the cause of their paralysis, the fact that they are paralyzed, and the fact that no treatment options for the paralysis exist. There also has to be a witness to the fact that the person is paralyzed. The person then visits the grotto and bathes in and drinks the water, and within hours a clear, observable change in the person's condition must occur. This change must result in complete and verifiable resolution of the condition. And finally, the person must return to be examined by the doctors at Lourdes in one year to confirm that the healing is lasting. By these criteria, more than seven thousand cases have been certified by the medical commission of Lourdes to be "unexplained healings."[1]

Each case takes an average of seven years to investigate, and these seven thousand certified cases are the end result of more than a million claims of healing that failed to meet the strict inclusion criteria. The Catholic Church has taken this rigorous examination even further and, in seventy of these cases, has publicly stated that a miracle has occurred with no explanation other than the waters of Lourdes. Many, but not all, of these cases involve people with cancer, all of whom have the imaging and pathology documentation demonstrating that they did have cancer, in many cases terminal cancer.

A 2012 paper published in the *Journal of the History of Medicine and Allied Sciences* undertook an ambitious review of reported healings at Lourdes and determined, "The least that can be stated is that exposures to Lourdes and its representations (Lourdes water, mental images, replicas of the grotto, etc.), in a context of prayer, have induced exceptional, usually instantaneous, symptomatic, and at best physical, cures of widely different diseases." The authors go on to describe Lourdes as having "considerable scientific interest" with the possibility of bringing about "new and effective therapeutic methods."[2]

The experiences people report are remarkably similar. People naturally enter the grotto with great hopes. Upon contact with the water, through either bathing or drinking, they feel a tingling sensation throughout their body. They frequently describe an unmistakable feeling of peace, relaxation, or comfort. After a few minutes, often to their surprise, whatever it was that ails them begins to feel different. Usually within hours it is clear that something has changed. For most people, it's not enough to resolve their illness, but for some—whether it resolves their illness or not—it is the most life-changing event in their lives.

It's worth noting that the experience people describe when they have had "success" at the Lourdes grotto is remarkably similar to what people report when they go to competent, honest, and true healers. Certainly, and for complex reasons, not everyone who goes to Lourdes or who goes to a true healer has a positive experience. But that some do is without a doubt, and anyone who claims to be a scientist must, at some point, come to grips with this. Just because mainstream medicine has no framework to understand how this healing could occur doesn't mean it doesn't occur. We need the humility to admit that our science is limited, as is our human understanding of these events.

During the late 1930s and into the years of the Second World War there was intense interest in developing nuclear weapons and nuclear energy technologies as an extension of our developing understanding of quantum and nuclear physics. One of the early repercussions of these early nuclear experiments was the "discovery" of the existence of various isotopes of hydrogen. Each element of the periodic table is defined by the number of protons it contains. The nucleus of each atom consists of positively charged protons and neutrons that have no charge. Both the protons and neutrons have equal weight and the weight is defined as one atomic unit. Swirling around this nucleus consisting of protons and neutrons are negatively charged electrons. Imagine planets revolving around the sun and that is the current conception of the electrons circling around the nucleus. Each atom in its resting state has a neutral charge, meaning the number of positively charged protons is equal to the number of negatively charged electrons. For example, hydrogen, the simplest and lightest atom, has one proton and one electron. Therefore it has a neutral charge, as do all atoms, and its atomic number is one. Atomic number is the sum of the protons (one) and neutrons (zero).

An isotope can be considered a variation on the theme of the atom. This means that in order to still be in the family of the original atom it must have the same number of protons as the original atom; in the case of hydrogen, the number is one. But the number of neutrons can change. Deuterium is one of the two known isotopes of hydrogen. It has one proton, so it is still "hydrogen," and it has one electron, so it is still electrically neutral, but it has one neutron instead of hydrogen's none. Its atomic number is therefore two (that is, one proton plus one neutron equals two).

Because deuterium is, in most respects, the same as hydrogen, it can form reactions in the same way, or at least in close to the same way, as hydrogen does. For our purposes, the most important reaction deuterium participates in is the formation of water. "Regular" water is H_2O, meaning it is the chemical bonding of two atoms of hydrogen with one atom of oxygen. Deuterium can also react in much the same way as hydrogen but instead forms D_2O. In the 1930s, when deuterium was first identified and recognized for its capacity to replace hydrogen in the formation of water, it was immediately clear that deuterium, so-called heavy water, is a naturally occurring substance. (Large quantities of pure heavy water can be produced through various nuclear reactions; it is called "heavy" because each deuterium is twice as heavy as hydrogen, therefore D_2O is heavier than H_2O.)

And while its biological role, if any, is still largely to be worked out, it was also clear pretty quickly that in high doses it is toxic to virtually all life-forms. If you water plants with it, or attempt to germinate seeds, or feed animals, they will fail to grow and soon will die. Pure heavy water is a strong biological poison.

It was then discovered that most naturally occurring nonsalt waters on the earth contain a small amount of naturally occurring D_2O. In other words, if you test the D_2O level of your local municipal water supply, the local stream, or a freshwater lake, it will typically test out to about 150 parts per million (ppm), a relatively small fraction. To picture this, if you imagine a liter of water, approximately one drop of the water is D_2O rather than H_2O. It should come as no surprise that our body fluids also contain D_2O at about the same level of 150 ppm.

D_2O, however, has many different physical properties than does H_2O. Chemically, it is a different molecule. For example, the freezing point of H_2O is 32°F (0°C). The freezing point of pure D_2O is 39.2°F (4°C). D_2O has a different density, the bond angles are different, and the maximum spectrum of light absorption is different. All in all, as we should expect, it is a different molecule with different biological and physical characteristics. The question is: Is that relevant to our health?

The thrust of this book is that the structure and integrity of intracellular water are fundamental to the health of our cells, tissues, and our entire organism. Both the structure and integrity impact cell division, transcription and translation of DNA for protein synthesis, energy generation, and the charge of the cell, and are the receptor mechanisms for everything from hormones and neurotransmitters to thoughts and emotions.

Our bodies have detoxification mechanisms to "purify" the intracellular matrix, we have natural medicines that affect the matrix, and we have just learned that if we drink certain water we may even be able to heal some of the worst diseases that afflict humankind.

So what factors in water itself impact its ability to form this perfect intracellular crystalline gel that is, I argue, the holy grail of health?

The first hint that high amounts of deuterium in the cells may interfere with human physiology came as a result of some Eastern European researchers who examined the water of isolated human communities that are known for their robust health and long lives.[3]

Because D_2O has a higher freezing point than H_2O, if you go into the mountains where water in the streams is coming from partially frozen glacial runoff, the water flowing under and around the frozen parts will be naturally lower in deuterium than the still frozen water. The way to picture this is to imagine taking a gallon jar of plain tap water and putting it in the freezer. At some point, there will be a fine layer of ice formed on the top of the still liquid water in the remainder of the jar. This fine layer of frozen water—the water that froze first—will have a higher concentration of deuterium in it than will the liquid water below. If you repeated this a dozen or so times you would end up with water that has had some part of its natural deuterium extracted: DDW. Glacial runoff is an example of the natural separation of the deuterium water from the hydrogen water.

While it is possible that other factors came into play to explain the long lives and complete absence of cancer in people who only consumed glacial runoff water, researchers were curious enough to see what would happen to animals, plants, and even people if they exclusively consumed a similar concentration of DDW. After all, water is by far the most abundant substance in our bodies and even though the ppm concentration of deuterium is low in our water, if we add up the total amount of deuterium in our bodies, it is approximately nine times (by weight) the amount of magnesium and four times (by weight) the amount of calcium. No one says magnesium and calcium have no role in our physiology or health.

These researchers found that deuterium has important biological functions. Or perhaps it is more accurate to say that hydrogen has many important biological functions and that the more we replace hydrogen with deuterium the more we interfere with these important biological functions. For example, the level of deuterium in the cell seems to be an important factor for stimulating cell division or mitosis. Without deuterium, the cells divide less readily; the more deuterium, the more rapid the cell division.[4] Of course, rapid, even uncontrolled cell division is one of the fundamental hallmarks of the cancer cell.

The researchers also found that hydrogen is the prime "ingredient" in the oxidative phosphorylation pathways that generate the ATP in the mitochondria. The more deuterium in the cell, the less hydrogen in the cell, the less efficient the generation of ATP becomes. Because ATP is necessary to properly structure intracellular water, an ATP deficiency is one of the primary hallmarks of the cancer process. Hydrogen deficiency then explains the biochemical basis of the mitochondrial dysfunction that is at the root of the Warburg effect. Finally and perhaps most importantly, deuterium is a different-sized and shaped molecule than hydrogen, and D_2O has a different size and shape than H_2O. Therefore, the intracellular gels formed by D_2O will be nowhere near as effective in organizing crucial cellular functions as H_2O is. Mistakes in division occur, the cellular charge becomes weak, the energy gradients in and around the cell weaken, and the receptive crystalline gels become distorted. The end result is an out of tune radio prone to various forms of sickness, including cancer.

This, of course, is *my* theory, but the basis of this theory is studies showing that if you take women with advanced breast cancer and give them standard oncology treatment or standard oncology treatment with the addition of DDW, the women who consume DDW do better. With the treatment protocols that have been worked out and "perfected" over the past fifty years and supported to the tune of many billions of dollars, the average life span of a typical patient with stage 4 breast cancer is still only twelve to thirty-one months.[5] If you simply add DDW, a little lower than occurs naturally in glacial runoffs, with no other interventions, the mean survival time for these same patients becomes fifty-two months.[6]

If you study women with early-stage breast cancer who are treated conventionally, their mean survival time is generally about 15 to 16 years. If you give these same women one six-month course of DDW, the mean survival time goes up to 18.1 years. If you instead give them two courses of DDW in the first five years, then their mean survival time goes up to 24.4 years.[7] It is certainly possible that I don't have a complete understanding of the entire mechanism by which DDW works to improve the prognosis for cancer patients. In fact, not only is that possible, I'm sure that is the case. The real issue, though, is when one gets results like this, published in peer-reviewed conventional scientific literature, why isn't this enough for the oncology community to conclude that while they may not understand the mechanism it's about time they looked into it?

In another study on the effect of DDW on cancer patients, researchers looked at men with prostate cancer. In the first part of the study they enrolled forty-four men with various stages of prostate cancer in a trial with twenty-two of the men receiving conventional treatment and the other twenty-two receiving DDW. The patients who received the DDW had a threefold net decrease in the volume of their prostate (meaning the prostate shrunk to more normal size), fifteen of the twenty-two had a decrease in the PSA level, and only two died. By contrast, in the conventional treatment group there was no net decrease in the volume of the prostate, only nine of the twenty-two men showed a decrease in PSA, and nine of the patients died. All of this reached statistical significance.[8] The researchers looked broadly at the mean survival time of prostate cancer patients treated with DDW compared to controls. Again, with similarly matched groups the mean survival time of the conventional treatment group was 15 to 20 months, whereas the group treated with DDW showed a mean survival time of 64.8 months.[9] Another source of information that can lead to new insights and new treatments for a variety of diseases is the publication of verified case reports on a particular therapy. In one, four patients with stage 4 lung cancer achieved a long-lasting remission as the result of treatment exclusively with DDW.[10]

We are not at a stage where we have a complete understanding of how DDW can have such a profound impact on the lives of cancer patients, but a clue comes from the world's foremost expert on water, Dr. Gerald Pollack. Dr. Pollack has undertaken an in-depth study of most of the famous healing waters of the world. One of his findings is that all of these waters, including some forms of DDW, have a characteristic peak of light absorption at the 270 nanometer (nm) band. This band is just below the wavelength of visible light, and the bond angles of the hydrogen (or deuterium) with the oxygen are of a characteristic angle. A good analogy is that the bond angles of the carbon atoms in a diamond are characteristic of the diamond and completely different than the bond angles found in a lump of coal. The elements that make up the substance are identical, it is their shapes that are altered, and clearly the shape is everything—at least everything that determines the characteristics of the substance. (If you don't believe me, give your fiancée a coal engagement ring and see what happens.) The tentative conclusion is that when the bond angles on the water have a peak absorption of 270 nm, then that water has the capacity to heal. If the water doesn't have a peak absorption of 270 nm, it can't and won't be a healing agent. There may be many ways to help the water achieve this structure, and lowering the deuterium levels in the water may be one. Having the water acted on by some external force, as in Lourdes, seems to be another.

The final piece of the DDW puzzle is: How do we explain the relationship between DDW and the ketogenic diet? Changing hydrogen for deuterium will naturally change the structure of whatever molecule this hydrogen/deuterium is incorporated into. Fats, due to their more delicate and precise configuration in space, are unable to incorporate deuterium into these large molecules. The deuterium simply won't fit into the shape needed for the fat molecule to form. Carbohydrates, on the other hand, easily incorporate deuterium into their less-precise folded structure. A good analogy in this case is that if your child is making a Lego sculpture out of the usual plastic Lego blocks and you decide to buy cheaper blocks made of paper, they look similar and kind of fit into the larger structure, but not exactly. Your child may be able to make very simple structures (carbohydrates), but when she tries to make more complex sculptures (fats), the cheap cardboard pieces simply collapse. Not only will your child be upset with you for getting cheap Lego pieces, she'll likely make you pay in the long run (with crankiness or demands for a bigger Lego set). Similarly, when you burn carbohydrates for fuel, you generate a lot of deuterium that will be incorporated in your body's water, and you will pay with poor health in the long run. On the other hand, if you burn fats as fuel, as in the ketogenic diet, you become naturally depleted of deuterium, with all the positive benefits that has for your intracellular water structure and your overall health.

Before I go on to explore the nature of forces that may be able to influence the water in our bodies and cells, we need to take one brief diversion into an interesting "supplement" that in some ways can be thought of as DDW in pill form. Then we can look at what is known about using water/etheric/negentropic forces directly to achieve this characteristic healing intracellular gel structure.

CHAPTER TEN

NADH

While there are many supplements that cancer patients use, sometimes to good effect, there is one supplement that stands out. My interest in NADH arises partly from its unique and interesting history in being helpful to people with many symptoms but also because its rationale for use corresponds to the rationale of this book. NADH, otherwise known as nicotinamide adenine dinucleotide hydride, is a natural substance found in our bodies. It is the biological form of hydrogen. In other words, when I talk about the role of hydrogen in our bodies, the reality is that there is no isolated molecular hydrogen to be found in any biological system. The hydrogen is bound in an almost infinite number of compounds, such as water, ATP, and every fat and protein in the body. NADH is the biological compound in our cells that delivers hydrogen to the mitochondria, where it is used to fuel oxidative phosphorylation and create ATP and intracellular water. In essence, we need oxygen, which we get through breathing, to combine with the hydrogen delivered from NADH to produce ATP and water. More importantly, NADH is often the limiting factor in the cellular production of ATP and water.

That is, we generally have enough of the other needed chemicals to produce ATP and water in our mitochondria; it is the NADH that limits these reactions. And, of course, if we become ATP deficient, many different disease states will arise.

The other important point, as Rudolf Steiner once suggested, is that the healthiest water in our cells is the water we create ourselves. If we drink water, and our intracellular water comes from this, then we will also ingest the many impurities, particularly deuterium, that are found in most sources of drinking water. In contrast, if our intracellular water comes largely from the water produced by the enzymatic reactions produced by oxidative phosphorylation, then the water will be a reflection of the chemical makeup of the reacting molecules. As far as I know, this has never been proven or even studied, but my guess is that, like fats, NADH is a complex molecule, only incorporates hydrogen in its structure, and is unable to substitute deuterium for hydrogen. If this is true then, as Steiner suggested, the water we create ourselves will be naturally low in deuterium and therefore similar to (but better than) drinking DDW.

We already know this is true for the fats; when they are metabolized in our cells, we produce DDW. It is likely also true that when we have adequate stores of NADH we naturally increase the amount of DDW in our cells, with all the corresponding health benefits I outlined in chapter 9.

Under the leadership of Dr. George Birkmayer, the Birkmayer Institute in Austria developed a reduced (hydrogenated) form of NADH and has been using it for decades, most notably in the treatment of patients with neurodegenerative disorders such as Parkinson's disease. At first, NADH could only be taken intravenously because the gastrointestinal tract will quickly degrade orally ingested NADH, but over time, the Birkmayer Institute was able to develop and patent NADH for oral use with similar therapeutic effects as the IV preparation. This allowed many more people to benefit from its use, which extends over a wide range of conditions in addition to neurodegenerative disorders.

Sometimes it is difficult for people, especially physicians, to understand how one medicine or intervention could treat such diverse conditions as Parkinson's disease, chronic fatigue syndrome, and cancer. The answer should be clear by now: The health of our cells, tissues, and therefore our bodies is based on the proper structuring of our intracellular water. This is a consequence of many factors, but two of the most important are the ability of our mitochondria to generate enough ATP to interact with our proteins to structure our water and the purity of the water. NADH interacts directly with both of these, making its mechanism of action, and its therapeutic effects, clear.

NADH is one of the most-studied molecules in molecular biology; thousands of citations refer to its various biological effects. Unfortunately, as far as I know there are no clinical trials that prove the value of the Birkmayer oral NADH protocol in cancer patients, but Dr. George Birkmayer has published a summary of his clinic's trials in cancer patients (see table 10.1).[1]

There are, of course, a lot of questions that remain unanswered, including repeatability, the absence of controlled studies, survival, and more. But a larger question remains: If credible

Table 10.1. NADH Trials with Cancer Patients

Type of Cancer	Number of Cases	Outcome, Tumor Regression	Outcome, Tumor Free
Prostate	17	10	7
Mammary	5	3	2
Glioblastoma	2	1	1
Non-Hodgkin's	3	2	1
Small-cell lung	3	1	2
Colon	4	1	3
Gastric	1	1	—
Pancreatic	1	1	—

physicians and researchers report these kind of results and we have numerous papers in peer-reviewed journals[2] that delineate the underlying mechanisms of how and why NADH has a positive effect on the cancer process, why isn't even 0.5 percent of our cancer budget urgently shifted to studying this medicine? To have the possibility of a natural, nontoxic substance, produced in our own bodies, with a plausible published mechanistic analysis on how and why it works, and yet for it to be completely ignored in the mainstream oncology community is baffling.

Dr. Birkmayer was gracious enough to share the stories of three cancer patients he treated in his clinic. The first was a forty-eight-year-old male with small-cell bronchial carcinoma diagnosed by magnetic resonance imaging (MRI) and biopsy who underwent radiation and chemotherapy for five months with no reduction of tumor mass. He started NADH, the tumor shrunk, and the tumor was undetectable a year following diagnosis. Twelve years later, he is alive, well, and still taking NADH. In another case, a fifty-six-year-old man with stage 2B anaplastic B-cell non-Hodgkin's lymphoma underwent unsuccessful chemotherapy and radiation. He refused further conventional treatment and started NADH. Two years later there was no evidence of the disease and the patient remains alive and well as of this writing. Finally, Dr. Birkmayer shared with me the story of a patient diagnosed with a tumor in the medulla (brain stem). The patient refused chemotherapy and started NADH. A CT scan six months later showed no detectable tumor. Six years later, the patient remains alive and well.

While these reports don't constitute "proof," the question remains: Since durable remissions such as these are so rare with cancer patients, why don't results like this merit a full-scale investigation into NADH, so that we might better support people struggling with cancer?

CHAPTER ELEVEN

Energetic Life Forces

I started this book by attempting to demonstrate that cancer is a cytoplasmic, rather than nuclear, disease. I then went on to look at the structure and nature of cytoplasm, attempting to show that it is, when healthy, structured (or gel phase) water. I then postulated that structured water is the essence or carrier of what has been called the life force, the etheric body (by Steiner), the negentropic force (by Schrödinger), even Chi (in Chinese medicine) or prana (in Ayurvedic medicine). In other words, life is water plus substance, raised into life. As esoteric as this may seem at first blush, I proposed that we all have an intuitive sense that there is more to life than inanimate substance. There is a force involved, a life force, and it can only work through the medium of water.

Good health means good crystalline gel formation in our cells. When we are in good health, we easily generate the energy we require, we charge our cells, we make the proper amount and type of proteins from our DNA, and thousands of other cellular functions proceed smoothly. When our gels are distorted, through poisons such as DDT, glyphosate, radiation, electromagnetic forces, aluminum in vaccines, or even destructive thoughts or emotions, we become more susceptible to disease. Healing, at its core, is the restoration of the integrity of the intracellular gels to their proper crystalline state. When I say "proper crystalline state," this refers to a state based on a general human blueprint that is individually modified, unique to each person. In other words, there is a "normal" intracellular gel configuration, but each of us modifies this, to some extent, to craft our unique individuality.

The interventions I've chosen to cover in this book have been used successfully for a variety of illnesses, including cancer, and each at its core—and each in its own way—is an attempt to restore the patient's intracellular gels to a more functional state. Gerson did this through detoxification and restoring Na+/K+ distribution across the cell membranes. DDW does this by providing the ill person with proper water, rather than heavy water, which is so problematic for many of our metabolic functions. NADH does this as the source of cellular hydrogen, thereby providing the raw material for the production of pure intracellular H_2O.

The final step, now that we have cleansed the gels, restored the ionic distribution inside to outside the cell, and provided the patient with good water, is to look directly at the nature of this life force and ask: How can we apply this force directly to the ill person? Is that possible and if so what does it look like? In other words, once we have clean cells and healthy water in our bodies, can we apply this force directly to "organize" the person back into a healthy, coherent whole? This is a question that has occupied some of the world's greatest mystics, thinkers, and healers for millennia. It is the most challenging kind of intervention for me to cover—there are a lot of things we just don't understand yet, as well as a lot of holes in the history and research literature—but I believe it is also one of the most promising avenues for us to pursue because it gets right to the heart of the intracellular matrix and the life force itself, and we would do well to investigate its promise as thoroughly as possible.

In this chapter, I am going to confine myself to the history of using this life force in modern times, primarily in Europe and

North America. Of course, working with life forces by no means started in Europe or North America in the twentieth century; in fact, this time frame doesn't even begin to cover the richness of the tradition. Life force is the essence of Chinese medicine, shamanic healing traditions, and European homeopathy. But for brevity and clarity, I am going to stick to recent western history and see what we can begin to discover there.

The first well-known person to suggest that using "energy," specifically electromagnetic fields in this case, to influence disease processes was probably Nikola Tesla. This seems to have been his greatest passion: how to harness the power of the electromagnetic fields to influence the course of disease. Although Tesla made many important discoveries that have borne fruit for the modern world, he never progressed very far in understanding how to use energy for healing. It was simply a seed planted that we have yet to harvest.

An obscure scientist named Royal Rife took things a bit further. Rife was a biologist, engineer, and inventor who lived near San Diego in the early twentieth century. By the mid-1930s he achieved recognition for his invention of a powerful new microscope with the resolution of modern electron microscopes, as well as the capacity to examine living tissues, cells, and organisms—unlike modern electron microscopes in which the tissue or cells or organisms must first be killed, fixed, and stained in order to be seen. Hundreds of times more powerful than any existing microscope available at that time, Rife's microscope opened up a new frontier of understanding microorganisms and living cells.

Unfortunately, what Rife observed under his microscope did not jibe with popular theories about the role of microbes in health and disease. At that time, as today, the germ theory of disease postulated that bacteria and viruses, each with its own life cycle and history, infect other organisms, like us, and cause disease. At the time, however, it was thought that the strep organism, for example, only could exist in its usual unicellular form, either in our throat or not, and if it did it would make us sick. What Rife saw under his microscope, however, was that some bacteria are *pleomorphic*, meaning they can assume different forms, and that the form they assume at any given time is a function of the conditions in which they exist. At times, some bacteria will assume an infective form, the form that is looked for and recognized by modern science. Under other conditions, the bacteria might form spores. Under yet other conditions an organism might assume a hyphal (or fungal) form. The form that developed depended on the growth conditions of the host or the medium in which the organism grew. As time went on, Rife was able to demonstrate this, using his microscope, to scores of interested and curious doctors, many of whom wrote testimonials supporting Rife's assertions.

The implications of Rife's findings for microbiology and medicine are enormous. Rife found he could manipulate the growing medium to determine the form. He showed that "infectious" disease does not so much come from the outside (although at some point you do have to be exposed), but is really a question of the "terrain," meaning the conditions in the body and mind, or maybe, more accurately, the water body. In other words, at a certain pH or oxygen tension, a spore form emerges. At a different pH or oxygen tension (or water structure), the hyphal form emerges. This is a revolutionary paradigm shift in how we understand and treat infectious disease, one that modern medicine has yet to fully understand or appreciate today.

Back in the 1930s, Rife was convinced that all patients with cancer had a particular kind of bacterial spore in their cells, particularly in the cancer cells. He believed he had found the cause of cancer, or at least the form of an organism that is always present in the cells of a person suffering from cancer. Although Rife missed the mark in this regard, I think he hit it spot on in his determination that the condition of the cell (in particular the condition of the gel matrix) influences, even determines, the form a microorganism will take. That is, we know now that every cell and every tissue type live in intimate connection with an almost unfathomable number of microorganisms—microorganisms that reside in breast tissue, in our brains, even under our eyelids—and that the form these organisms take is largely influenced by the surrounding environment in which they reside.

Rife's next step, as an electrical and mechanical engineer, was to expose the spore forms found in cancer cells to a "plasma field" that would destroy the organisms even in their resistant spore form. He developed a device—a device that is, as far as I can tell, impossible to re-create or fully understand—that reliably destroyed the spore form of the "cancer bacteria" in Petri dishes. He could see this using his microscope. Other doctors testified to seeing this as well. Then, he took the crucial step of exposing animals with cancer to his plasma fields. He reported high cure rates in the infected animals.

The next step, of course, was to use his techniques in people suffering from cancer. At this point, an understandable skepticism arises (if it hasn't arisen already). It's hard to understand exactly what Rife was doing and we don't fully understand the energy field he was using. But I nevertheless find his work significant and worth trying to understand because what we can reasonably state is that when he and others saw this spore form—whatever it ultimately was—they could find an energetic frequency that would "explode" it, and when they did, animals (and, in some cases, people) seemed to recover. Rife's work is more murky than I would like, but it is also one of the cleanest examples of using energy to quickly eradicate cancer, and on that basis I feel his work merits acknowledgment and additional research in order to better understand its potential.

If we don't really understand what Rife's plasma field actually was and reports about it lie in the murky past, and the cases, even if true, are passed off as anecdotal, how can this become any kind of basis for rigorous science? Some physicians working with Rife at the time were aware of the controversial nature of the work. Because of this, they formed a commission consisting of five physicians and pathologists from around the country to supervise and document Rife's experiment with sixteen terminally ill cancer patients. The trial reports claim that fourteen of the sixteen terminally ill cancer patients treated by the Rife plasma device were cured.

Arthur W. Yale, MD, remarked, "Mr. Rife has succeeded in finding a vibratory rate which will kill the different invading organisms of the body.... Having used this apparatus for almost two years, the writer has had the satisfaction of witnessing the disappearance of every malignant growth, where the patient has remained under treatment."[1]

Another doctor remarked, "I put my hand on his stomach which was just one solid mass, just about what I could cover with my hand, somewhat like the shape of a heart. It was absolutely solid! And I thought to myself, well, nothing can be done for that. However, they gave him a treatment with the Rife frequencies and in the course of time over a period of six weeks to two months, to my astonishment, he completely recovered."[2]

Robert J. Houston, MD, was a colleague of Rife's who defended the value of anecdotal cases such as these in the search for the causes of and treatments for cancer. "In cancer, case studies have a greater degree of validity than in other diseases. In cancer, the rate of spontaneous remission is extremely low, so low that it is virtually zero. Therefore, if you have just a few cases, basically if you have two cases, you have something that is solid. So I consider what is being dismissed as anecdotal evidence to be, in cancer, actually an impressive area of evidence, because you have much more detail in case studies than you can in a clinical trial."[3]

Interestingly, even though the focus of Rife's treatment was using the plasma field device on the patient until he could see that the bacterial spores were eradicated, Rife remarked about the nature of his treatment: "In reality, it is not the bacteria themselves that produce the disease, but the chemical constituents of these microorganisms enacting upon the unbalanced cell metabolism of the human body that in actuality produce the disease. We also believe if the metabolism of the human body is perfectly balanced or poised, it is susceptible to no disease."[4]

My interpretation of the story of Royal Rife is that there is evidence that terminally ill cancer patients had their disease reversed as a direct result of being exposed to the plasma field of the Rife device. It seems that by using the microscope he developed with its resolution powers far exceeding those of the usual microscopes at that time, he could visually see when the organisms he associated with cancer were removed and therefore the patient would be able to recover. And, finally, even though the focus of his work was on visually documenting the pleomorphic bacterial life-forms, he believed that it was the intracellular environment in the patient that allowed these cancer spores to develop. For me, if we substitute the words *plasma field* for *life/etheric/negentropic force*, Rife and I are talking about the same thing.

As time went on, Rife's work came under scrutiny of the medical authorities and he was ordered to stop his work. The field of electromagnetic medicine in oncology and the use of plasma wave technology for cancer patients went dormant and only resurfaced with the work of a Frenchman named Antoine Prioré in the 1960s.

Primarily an inventor, physicist, and engineer, Prioré developed a plasma ray device that was possibly the first to use conjugated waves and that—as I understand it—allows the healer to direct the energy of the apparatus to resonate with the energy of the patient. Think of it as a tuning device and the patient as a piano. If you can find the precise resonant frequency, the tuning fork will accentuate the sound of the note you are striking. Whereas Rife used destructive frequencies to rid the body of the spore form of the bacteria he saw as being involved in the cancer process, Prioré used resonant frequencies of the plasma field to support the life force of the patient. Both, according to eyewitness reports, were able to reverse cancer in animal and human subjects.

With Prioré's work, there were numerous reports of healing of cancer in animals, especially leukemia, over the course of two decades, but few reports with human subjects. And as with Rife, there was conflict with the French medical authorities and Prioré's work was halted just before large clinical trials with human patients could be performed.

Before I turn to modern "energy devises," I want to reiterate that the intention of this book has never been to offer a finished theory or complete treatment plan. My intention is to point out that after fifty years and billions of dollars having been spent pursuing one particular view of cancer, it is past time to both reverse course and widen our horizons. If even 1 percent of the total cancer expenditures in the last fifty years had gone to studying the Rife plasma device, the Prioré protocols, DDW, and other interventions I have discussed in this book, imagine how much further along we might be today. (Not to mention what would have happened if we had taken half of those resources and devoted them to producing a clean, healthy, and safe environment.) It should be no surprise that a solo general practitioner working in a small practice in San Francisco who has spent his entire career being thwarted by the medical establishment attempting to access therapies that might help patients survive and mitigate their suffering doesn't have the answer to cancer. The question should be: Why haven't any promising leads been pursued by a medical establishment that claims to be looking out for our best interest, but is so clearly not? I believe everyone should be asking this question—and demanding an answer.

I want to answer my own question with a story from my childhood. As a child I was fascinated by stories of Native Americans and other indigenous peoples. When I heard about the conquest of the American continent by Europeans, I was tormented by it. Why couldn't the Europeans even take *some* of the continental United States and leave a decent part for the Native Americans? Why did "we" need it all? No one I know has ever had any reasonable answer to this simple question.

Then, about ten years ago, I was reading a passage in a book by Derrick Jensen referring to the US Army manual, describing how to handle the issue of prisoner exchanges. The US Army had a problem: When one of its soldiers was captured by Native Americans and it came time to exchange him for a captured Native American, the US soldier would refuse to return to his army regimen. On the other hand, Native American captives would bolt as soon as possible to be reunited with their tribe. The manual describes various techniques to lure the soldiers back to their regimen, including promises of money, women, and food, but these strategies rarely worked. These "unredeemed captives" often found that life was better with their Native American captors.

For me, this explains the reason "we" took, and take, it all. It explains why the cancer establishment, to survive, must wipe out any possible options for understanding or treating the disease. For it is clear to everyone that leaving even one small option will blow the cover off the whole operation. Once word gets out, the emperor will be found to have no clothes. Members of the establishment understand this all too well. They must have it all.

Over the course of more than two decades, I have investigated or used at least a dozen "devices" that claim to be modern equivalents of the Rife or Prioré devices. The manufacturer typically offers information about the interaction of the devices' energy with the patient to demonstrate that its device is the state of the art in modern energy healing. These devices include modern Rife machines, pulsed electromagnetic field devices, and biophoton devices that make use of various energy frequencies or colors to provide healing. I have seen and used sound-healing devices, color therapy devices, and devices that use "phase-conjugation" waves to create a heightened energy state in the sick human being. I have seen positive effects from all of these, but I have not seen the kind of convincing evidence that would lead me to proclaim one or the other as *the* state-of-the-art healing device.

At the same time, the re-creation of a safe, effective energy device, one that can directly work with the negentropic life force, should be one of the highest priorities for the medical research community. This is the holy grail of medicine, one that could lead to an untold reduction of suffering at little cost. An effective modern version of the Rife device would be the biggest breakthrough possible in medicine, one I haven't seen happen, but eagerly await.

The bottom line is this: Certain forms of ambient energy are not only good for us but necessary for life. For example, the energy from the sun is a crucial ingredient for almost all life-forms on earth. Similarly, the energy from the earth itself, now being studied as "earthing" or "grounding," shows that the earth's energy is imperative for all life-forms on earth, including humans. Another source of "good" energy is the energy "emitted" by human beings themselves, which is especially concentrated in the palms of our hands. This beneficial energy may at least partially explain the benefits we feel from holding the hands of our loved ones, or from such things as the "laying on of hands" or Reiki.

Some of Dr. Gerald Pollack's experiments into the flow of water also demonstrate this good energy. Any hydrophilic tube immersed in a beaker of water will create a small negatively charged gel layer lining the tube. This means that there will also be free protons—the corresponding positive charges liberated when the gels are formed—that go into the liquid water in the center of this tube. These positive ions repel each other and initiate flow within the tube.

If you put this beaker of water with the suspended tube in a lead box, thereby shielding out all forms of energy, the flow will cease. If you then take the beaker out of the box and expose it to sunlight, the flow will resume. This is because the sun is the energy source for the formation of the gel phase water lining the tube. If you put the beaker on the earth, flow increases. If you put your hands on the beaker, flow also increases. Even if you put your dog or cat next to the beaker, flow will increase.

On the other hand, if you want to see the effect of Wi-Fi energy on living systems, just put your cell phone next to the beaker and watch the flow cease. Non-native electromagnetic forces directly inhibit our ability to form crystalline gels in our cells. As a result, no cellular functions will work properly. Non-native electromagnetic forces destroy life by destroying the basis of life, which is the intracellular gel.

I often think that the field of energy healing, be it Rife machines, spiritual healers, Reiki, or the like, would be well served if it could only realize that the energy it is tapping into will work only insofar as it facilitates the creation of healthier gels. I am also convinced that this is the fundamental basis of homeopathy. The patient describes her condition (some abnormality of intracellular gel) and the homeopath matches this with the "frequency" of the remedy. The resonance of these two united forces creates the possibility of healing. This may also be why being around people whose "energy" we experience as negative has such dire consequences for our health.

Many times in my life, as I grappled with a seemingly unsolvable problem, I turned my attention to wondering whether I was asking the wrong question. After decades of looking for *the* healing energy device, it struck me recently that I have been overlooking the most sophisticated, energetic healing device ever created: human consciousness. Quantum physics, the area of science at the forefront of understanding this new biology I speak of, is clear that human consciousness is the fundamental force from which our universe is created. As Henry Stapp, physicist at the Lawrence Berkeley National Laboratory, remarked, "We have known for almost a century that this theoretical creation of the human mind called 'classical physics' is a fiction of our imagination."[5]

In other words, a universe that consists only of billiard balls, of lifeless matter as proposed by Descartes and that forms the basis of our modern medicine, is a fictitious construct of our imagination. Or, as French quantum physicist Bernard d'Espagnat put it, "The doctrine that the world is made up of objects whose existence is independent of human consciousness turns out to be in conflict with quantum mechanics."[6] That is to say, direct experimental evidence has demonstrated that the theory of a universe composed only of "stuff" is not actually supported by the evidence. Physicist Max Planck remarked, "I regard consciousness as fundamental. I regard matter as derivative from consciousness. We cannot get behind consciousness."[7]

The question must be, then: How do we harness the incredible, creative power of human consciousness in the service of healing our most insidious diseases? While there may not be a clear or easy answer to this question, my suggestion is that the best place to look is in the confluence of prayer and meditation. These are the thousands of years old techniques used to harness the power of human consciousness in the service of human and universal well-being. And, as so eloquently pointed out by Stephan A. Schwartz and Larry Dossey, MD, if prayer were a new medicine patentable by our current medical institutions, it would be hailed as the greatest breakthrough in medical history.[8]

The Heart of Centering Prayer, described in detail in the book *The Heart of Centering Prayer* by Cynthia Bourgeault, is a simple, but profound, technique to access the power of human consciousness.[9] It does so by connecting the mind to the heart, which, as I described in my book *Human Heart, Cosmic Heart*, should be acknowledged as the center of human consciousness. The prayer is designed to help you move past the process of thinking, the domain of the brain, into the experience of knowing, a process that I would link with the heart. *Thinking*—I prefer to call it *deciding*—is when you decide to pursue a career because the pay and benefits are appealing. *Knowing* is when you feel called to a profession because of an inner sense of your own destiny. Deciding is when you choose a life partner because it's time to settle down. Knowing is when you realize your destiny is inexorably linked with that of the person you love. Deciding often comes about through fear, fear of not making a living, being alone, or that if you don't do conventional therapy you will die. Knowing comes from a place of freedom, a place in which you know that the choice you make could be no other.

A friend of mine, an oncologist who helped develop Abnoba viscum mistletoe therapy, which is now widely used in European oncology, had every new cancer patient, as long as time would allow it, gather information from as many different types of practitioners as possible. He wanted them to present their story to at least one conventional oncologist, to healers, herbalists, and mistletoe practitioners such as himself, and to their trusted family doctor. Then, once this information had been gathered, he asked them to take at least a week and either meditate or pray about their course of action. The information gathering was a way to connect with the patient's deciding activity, centered in the brain. Once they had done this, they could go deeper and connect with their inner path, a process more connected with their heart. It was his experience that patients who chose a therapy, whichever one they chose, had better outcomes when the choice came from the heart. Making heart-centered choices is when the miracles, such as those I describe in this book, tend to happen.

The Heart of Centering Prayer will help facilitate this process. Paradoxically, as the prayer will show, it comes not through an active engagement with your heart, but once you have moved past the normal thinking activity that occupies so much of our consciousness. Once we start to tame this "monkey brain," as it is called in meditation circles, through a process akin to grace, this universal life force can begin to reveal itself. When decisions are made from this position of knowing, worlds will open to you that had been hidden before. It's not a therapy for cancer, or any other disease, but it will help you open to the powerful world of unseen forces and to a way of knowing and proceeding that is particularly valuable to those confronting serious illness.

The fact that meditation or prayer is not a therapy per se is perhaps exactly the point. Cancer, as I have outlined, is a complex disease. Perhaps one of these components is that humans are asleep to their true nature. Rather than attempting to eradicate disease, what is urgently needed is for us to wake up, to recognize the energetic and spiritual nature of our being, and let this awakening reorganize, rearrange, and heal our physical organism.

PART III

Practical Steps Forward for Individuals

CHAPTER TWELVE

A Basic Cancer
Therapy Framework

If you look at the history of medicine, particularly European medicine, over the past several centuries, you find two diametrically opposed views of the philosophy of treatment. What we think of as conventional, allopathic medicine is completely diagnosis-oriented and cares not a whit about the experience of the patient. I don't mean this in a derogatory way. I simply mean that the goal is to treat everyone with strep throat the same regardless of their age, symptoms, or individual tendencies. Doctors are taught to find the diagnosis, and then match that with the treatment that corresponds to that diagnosis. Everyone with strep gets penicillin (or some other antibiotic), everyone with pancreatic cancer gets gemcitabine (some get surgery depending on whether it's possible), and everyone with depression gets Prozac or a similar antidepressant. It doesn't matter who you are, why you got these conditions, or what your opinion is about this therapy.

In contrast, traditional or classical homeopathy cares *only* about the experience of the patient. One person with strep throat will get one remedy, another person with strep throat will get a different remedy for the same disease. Homeopathy is entirely based on the experience of the person. The treatment strategy is to match up the experience of the person with the symptom picture that is caused when you ingest a certain, often poisonous, substance. For example, a person ingesting belladonna will get dilated pupils, feel fearful, and often have a fever and a sore throat. If a person presents with those symptoms, belladonna is their remedy. Whether or not the patient has strep is irrelevant.

There could not be two fundamentally different ways of looking at medicine than homeopathy and allopathic medicine.

Anthroposophical medicine bridges this gap. There are typical medicines for each disease, but a healer always tailors the therapy to the experience of the patient. As we will discuss, this comes into play in our use of mistletoe because a cancer patient who is thin, with a desiccated appearance, may do better with mistletoe from a pine tree, and a round, warm person might be best treated with mistletoe from apple trees. Some cancer patients have a prominent history of exposure to environmental toxins. They would be well served with aggressive detoxification. For others, their story is more one of emotional withdrawal and trauma; for these patients a strategy that uses more gentleness and warmth must be employed. Anthroposophical medicine is an attempt to merge the "reality" of the conventional diagnosis with an in-depth sensitivity for the patient sitting in front of you. It is also, therefore, difficult to make up simple frameworks with regard to treatment (i.e., treat this disease with this medicine). Every person is unique; every prescription, therefore, must be individualized. That is the true art of medicine.

The majority of conventionally trained doctors are unequipped to do such individualized medicine, mostly because they have never even heard of such a thing. But when the doctor is aware of both sides and has an in-depth understanding of the nature of the disease, combined with a sensitivity for the human being sitting in front of her, that is precisely when the magic and the "miracles" of healing happen. We need more healers who are able to work in this manner and right now we don't have them— our health care system doesn't support, or even tolerate, them.

In the framework I outline in this chapter, the personalized prescription is left out. This should be clear from the outset. There is no intention for my framework to replace the care of a knowledgeable physician skilled in the art of medicine. This framework is simply meant as a place to start for a patient suffering from cancer. It is based on my review of the relevant medical literature, my personal experience with my patients, and my hopes for the future of medicine and better outcomes. It may also give people ideas they can then suggest to open-minded doctors as possible avenues to explore. But fundamentally it is a simplified framework for an area of life that doesn't really lend itself to frameworks. We are dealing with the life of a human being and all the complexity that entails. This should never be forgotten.

In addition to suggesting that my readers find a practitioner who is well versed in the holistic treatment of cancer patients along the lines I am outlining here, I feel it is also important to point out that in my more than thirty-five years of treating cancer patients, the majority of my successful patients have used a combination of surgery and the interventions I discuss in this book. All of the mistletoe-treated patients I presented have used this combination of surgical "debulking" followed by the mistletoe therapy. Although Rudolf Steiner at one point suggested that, in the future, mistletoe should be able to replace the knife, surgical intervention is generally the standard around the world in mistletoe use. The original patients treated with the Rife device and Birkmayer's NADH, and many people using the Gerson therapy, have been successful forgoing any surgical intervention. There is a significant body of research suggesting that surgically removing the primary tumor facilitates distant metastasis, exactly what we don't want. So while it is clear that the tumor is not the disease— cancer is a cytoplasmic dysfunction—it should nevertheless be recognized that is a lot to ask of the body to resorb a large number of cancerous cells. My experience suggests that surgically removing whatever can be safely removed, followed by the implementation of the therapies suggested here, produces the best outcome.

As for the use of conventional chemotherapy along with this program, this combination is something each person should work out with his oncologist. At times, this seems to be the best solution; at other times the chemotherapy is so toxic that the gentle approach outlined in this chapter is simply ineffective. This decision simply has to be made on a case-by-case basis.

For each medicine I cover in this chapter, appendix A (page 163) offers options for sourcing it. Unfortunately, in some cases, usually due to regulatory concerns, there are few if any good options. I have chosen to include them anyway because it is my sincere hope that in the near future Americans will be allowed freedom of choice, including an availability of natural medicines that does not exist at this time.

Finally, my goal with treatment has always been to emphasize things that people can do themselves without the need for prescriptions or expert advice. This is not always possible or even advisable, but as much as possible my goal is to empower people and to provide individuals with low-cost options that can be used safely and effectively at home. For this reason, I have avoided protocols that require intravenous medicines and other clinic- or hospital-based interventions. It's not that these interventions, such as hyperthermia and IV vitamin C, aren't useful. It's that right now they are not possible for the vast majority of people. With that introduction, here are the basics of the program.

Diet

The basic dietary principles for this cancer therapy framework are similar to the dietary principles I have laid out in my previous books. That is, first and foremost, this diet is quality-based. By quality, I mean everything from the soil in which the food is grown to the harvesting techniques, storage, food preparation, and even the emotional state of the people growing, processing, and preparing the food. Quality means knowing where your food comes from, knowing your farmer, and visiting the farms where your food is grown. Hopefully one of the gardens that grows your food is your own.

Another way to say this is that no one who has successfully used diet to heal from a serious condition ate eggs from sick, battery cage–confined chickens. All of your food must be of the best quality. This means pastured animal products, biodynamic or beyond organic plant foods, and pure water. *Nourishing Traditions* by Sally Fallon should serve as your food guide, and the work of the Weston A. Price Foundation can provide you with valuable information about where to obtain and how to prepare the foods. With this general information there are a number of specific points that people with cancer should bear in mind.

Macronutrients

Macronutrients refers to the amount of fat, protein, and carbohydrates you eat. The general principle is to look for the best-quality fats—grass-fed ghee or butter, coconut oil, and olive oil—in unlimited amounts guided by your taste and instincts. Your protein consumption should be moderate, about the size of a deck of cards twice per day. Carbohydrates should be counted and limited. Each person should strive to consume 20 to 30 grams of carbohydrates, total, in all their food, twice per day. There are many good books and guidelines explaining how to count carbs in common foods. Many people will feel fatigue initially at this low level of carbohydrate consumption; if so, the best strategy is to slowly reduce to this amount and let your body adjust to getting fuel from the fats. This will usually happen in about six to eight weeks.

Timing

The goal of timing is to go through periods of the day and month where you are in ketosis, which means that you will be burning fat as fuel instead of glucose. Ketosis has many proven benefits for cancer patients, and for most people. The process of ketosis burns your own excess fat, reduces inflammation, increases cerebral blood flow, and stimulates apoptosis, one of the most important ways your body rids itself of cancer cells. The simplest and most practical way to time your eating for ketosis is to restrict eating to a six-hour period each day and do water-only fasts for the other eighteen hours. Practically speaking, it is best to eat one good meal at 8 a.m., a second good meal at 2 p.m., and then only have water between 2:30 p.m. and 8 a.m. the next morning. You can vary the timing to suit your needs, but this rhythm of six hours of food and about eighteen hours of fasting is a good long-term strategy.

In addition, unless you are underweight, a three-day water-only fast once a month is helpful for intensifying the ketosis and supporting all the health benefits nutritional ketosis provides. Again, there are good books that explain in detail how to do various forms of water-only fasting. The only caveat is that if you are underweight or losing weight, I suggest you skip the three-day fast.

Bone Broth

Two to six cups of bone broth per day is an important part of a sound cancer diet. Cells use the proteins in bone broth as the nidus for structuring water inside the cells. Bone broth proteins are made of different amino acids than are meat proteins. These amino acids are often deficient in western diets, leading to weak support structures and poor ability to create healthy intracellular gels.

All of the bones used in making broth should be organic and pasture-raised, as commercial hay and feed are often heavily contaminated with glyphosate. *Nourishing Broth*, by Sally Fallon, goes into detail about the history of bone broth along with practical strategies for how to make it at home.

Vegetables

Vegetables are the therapeutic part of traditional diets. Fats and proteins are used to build structure, and plant nutrients provide the chemicals that help us prevent and treat disease. As such, each person should eat a wide variety of plants every day. This strategy fits perfectly with the restricted carbohydrate framework I am presenting. In addition to the usual garden vegetables, you should attempt to include a variety of nutrient-concentrated wild and perennial vegetables, including plants like wild ramps, artichokes, wild greens, Gynura procumbens (Okinawan spinach), and many others. You should also eat medicinal plants each day, including ashitaba (either fresh or one to two teaspoons of powder per day), burdock root (either fresh or one to two teaspoons of powder per day), and turmeric (two to four tablespoons per day)—preferably heat these plants or powders in a pan with ghee, then sauté the rest of the dish on top, and finish it with freshly ground black pepper. Finally, you should drink two to four cups of brewed chaga tea daily, along with two droppers of an alcoholic chaga extract twice per day to make sure you get both the water- and fat-soluble components of chaga. (Alcohol draws out fat-soluble nutrients.)

One of the easiest ways to include these vegetables and powders in your diet is to start each day with bone broth soup. To make it, heat a generous amount of grass-fed ghee in the pan, and dissolve one to two tablespoons of turmeric powder until dispersed. Add three to seven different vegetables and sauté them until they are soft. Add the homemade bone broth. Bring to a boil, then turn the heat down to a simmer. Add vegetable powders and some powdered sea vegetables, simmer a few more minutes, then ladle into a bowl with a tablespoon of naturally fermented miso and natto. This is one of the most satisfying breakfasts I eat, and one that I have eaten almost every day for the last three years.

Ferments

Everyone, especially everyone suffering from poor health, should eat fermented foods every day. This includes a variety of foods from all categories, including fermented dairy products, such as yoghurt, kefir, cottage cheese, cheese; soybeans (miso, natto); meat; vegetables; fruits; and grains. Naturally fermented vegetables, especially sauerkraut, are particularly important. (Add a dollop of sauerkraut to your finished breakfast soup.) Include a small amount of something fermented at every meal to aid in digestion. Fermented foods are found in virtually all traditional cultures and cuisines around the world.

With your diet, be creative, enjoy your food, experiment, share meals with friends and loved ones, and get to know the people who grow and process your food. This will enrich your life in an untold number of ways.

Supplements

There are a number of supplements I have discussed in this book that are a part of this cancer therapy framework.

Quinton Isotonic Seawater

The first supplement I suggest to all people with cancer, or almost any other serious disease, is Quinton isotonic seawater. As I suggested in chapter 4, not only is this the best source of all needed minerals, but also it essentially acts like a "structured" water supplement. It comes in either liter bottles or individual packets and the usual starting dose is thirty milliliters per day, divided into two equal doses.

NADH

The second important supplement for supporting people with any kind of mitochondrial or energy dysfunction is NADH. With NADH, the brand is crucial. Only the Birkmayer company has an oral form that is fully functional. The usual starting dose is eight tablets twice per day of the Rapid Energy form of NADH on an empty stomach. Let it dissolve thoroughly in your mouth. After a few months at this dose, you can reduce the dose to four tablets of the Rapid Energy NADH twice per day for the next six months.

Strophanthus Extract

I also recommend *Strophanthus* extract. The seed extract is the only effective form; homeopathically prepared *Strophanthus* doesn't appear to be effective and pure chemical ouabain seems to have little if any effect. The dose is one capsule three times a day on an empty stomach.

Melatonin

Another supplement that everyone confronting cancer should consider taking is melatonin. In Rudolf Steiner's cosmology he repeatedly discussed his concept of our four "bodies," the details of which can be found in many of his writings and in my book *The Fourfold Path to Healing*. He taught that we are made not just of a physical body, but also an etheric or water body, an astral or air body, and an ego or warmth body. This book has been mostly about a description of the role and function of our water or etheric body and how this body interacts with our physical substance in health and disease.

Another of Steiner's fundamental teachings is that when we sleep or when we are in a coma, we retain our substance (i.e., the physical body), we are still alive so the etheric or water body remains, but the soul (consciousness) and ego (self-consciousness) leave the etheric-physical "complex." This separation allows for the etheric and physical body to heal unimpeded by the demands of our feeling and thinking lives. This concept comes through in our common language as we refer to a person in a coma as being "a vegetable" or in a " vegetative" state; in other words they are a plant as far as the composition of their bodies is concerned. The important point here is not the jargon, but that

141

during sleep our water body is unimpeded in its interaction with our physical body and that this is when healing takes place. This concept is also currently being recognized in mainstream medicine as we learn more about the importance and healing power of sleep.[1]

Unquestionably the physical substance most associated with sleep is the hormone melatonin. Melatonin is produced not only in the brain, but in other tissues such as the intestines, thymus, bone marrow, and the cells of our immune system. It is produced primarily when we are asleep—more abundantly when we sleep in a completely dark room—and its synthesis is inhibited by exposure to non-native electromagnetic fields. Most of us produce little if any melatonin after the age of fifty, and people who have age-related illnesses will often experience relief when they replenish it. Some of the conditions for which melatonin has shown benefit include infections, cardiovascular disease such as hypertension, oxidative stress, Alzheimer's and neurodegenerative diseases, macular degeneration, and cancer. Melatonin accomplishes its effect through various biochemical pathways, including immune stimulation, increase of apoptosis, protection against radiation damage, telomerase inhibition, and many others. Melatonin supplementation has been shown to improve survival, potentiate chemotherapy, and stimulate tumor regression.[2] There is not a single cancer therapy parameter that melatonin supplementation has not been shown to improve in the medical literature.

The literature on the role of melatonin in improving cancer parameters is robust and convincing. What is left out of this literature is that melatonin is the hormonal, physical correlate, or marker, of the activity of an unimpeded water or etheric body that only happens during sleep. As such, its use is justified in the approach I am suggesting, which is a healing approach to the water body of the human being.

The most effective dose of melatonin for non-cancer-related illnesses seems to be much larger than the doses commonly used.

The following dose suggestions reflect optimal physiological states. For noncancer the dose is 180 milligrams before bed; with cancer prevention or therapy, the optimal dose is probably 60 milligrams four times per day before breakfast, lunch, dinner, and bedtime. As with all therapies, dosing of melatonin should be done in consultation with your treating physician or oncologist.

Water

The ideal water for general consumption should be toxin- and additive-free, low-deuterium water that is delivered through naturally vortexing channels. Ideally, instead of expensive individual systems, communities would come together to provide water to everyone. Unfortunately, that ideal situation is far from the reality for most people. Instead we drink water that is high in deuterium and full of toxic components such as chloramines, fluorides, residuals from pharmaceutical drugs, and a host of other unwanted substances. Obviously, this is something that needs to be addressed by anyone seeking to heal from a chronic disease. At this point, I know of no perfect options. There are a few companies that sell water that has been processed to contain lower amounts of deuterium, and these are the waters that have produced the beneficial results I discussed in chapter 9.

There are two common strategies in the use of DDW. The first is to gradually reduce the amount of deuterium in all drinking water over a matter of months. The second is to start with very depleted water (25 ppm) and essentially let this water dilute the level of deuterium in our cells. My preference is the first approach: All the water you drink for the first two months is about 125 ppm. You can then lower it to 105 ppm for two months, 75 ppm for two months, and then finally 60 ppm for six months. Some specialists advocate testing the levels of deuterium in your tissues and letting those levels guide the therapy. Theirs is a newer approach and one that should be thoroughly investigated.

There are companies that sell glacial runoff from the Rocky Mountain range that contains about 135 ppm deuterium. It is bottled in plastic, which is far from ideal, and the water is left to sit in the bottles for months, meaning it has probably lost all its structure by the time it is consumed. Furthermore, lowering the deuterium content to 135 ppm might not be enough to be therapeutically relevant.

There is a desperate need for the technology to safely produce DDW for all communities. It should be made in all of the above-mentioned ppm levels, put through a vortex, and distributed cheaply in glass bottles. Until then, it is best to contact the companies I provide in appendix A (page 163) that are able to provide DDW and instruct people in its use.

Mistletoe

Of all the interventions I describe in this book, mistletoe is the one for which it is most crucial to find a practitioner with extensive experience in its use. I started using mistletoe with patients in the late 1980s and have treated hundreds of patients with it since then. As with anything worth studying, the more you know about it, the more questions you'll have. My overall impression of mistletoe is that we are too meek in its use. Mistletoe will produce a significant local reaction to its usual administration if administered via subcutaneous injection. And it can and will produce a strong febrile response if that is the desired goal. My experience is that in order to see a benefit, you have to stimulate a visible and clear response. For the past five years, I have only used the Helixor form of mistletoe injections because Helixor mistletoe seems to produce the most reliable responses as well as the best clinical outcomes.

In Germany and most of Europe, there are many different preparations of mistletoe available. The one that is the most widely used and studied is Iscador, a type of fermented mistletoe extract, but many companies have experimented with various preparations to increase its efficacy. Some preparations concentrate the active ingredients, the viscotoxins and mistletoe lectins. There are also nonfermented varieties, and varieties from different trees, all of which concentrate different active ingredients, and even some preparations that add purified mistletoe lectins back into the ampules.

Helixor sells an unfermented mistletoe preparation made from mistletoe growing on either the fir tree, the apple tree, or the pine tree. Each of these mistletoe products has different properties and is indicated for different kinds of cancer (and different types of people). Helixor has a website that explains the properties of each type of mistletoe, as well as a program in which any patient or physician anywhere in the world can ask the Helixor staff physicians for guidance on which mistletoe is suitable and the guidelines for its use. I suggest every patient and every physician new to the use of mistletoe should take full advantage of their expertise in guiding your therapy.

Generally, when a physician is confronted with a cancer patient, the process is to first match the site of the primary tumor with the type of mistletoe that complements that tumor type. For prostate cancer, for example, it is the mistletoe that grows on fir trees. The patient is then started on fir tree mistletoe injections subcutaneously in the abdomen, a process easily learned by virtually all patients, three times per week. Starting with series 1, you gradually increase the dose until the mistletoe produces either a localized redness (at least silver dollar–sized) or a fever. The dose remains at this level until the patient stops reacting, at which time you increase the dose another increment. This three-times-per-week injection strategy creates a kind of dialogue between the patient's immune system and the mistletoe. We increase the strength until the immune system tells us it has been stimulated. We keep the dose there until no reaction happens, then we increase again. In this slow step-wise fashion, we increase from 1 milligram of the weakest fir mistletoe up to 150 milligrams of the strongest pine mistletoe. We always continue with the same tree until no more reactions occur with that form of mistletoe. In this way, over the years we have an ongoing interaction and dialogue between the immune reactivity of the patient and the mistletoe.

There are, of course, many nuances that arise during the course of the therapy. This is where it is crucial to have the support of an experienced physician, as well as a dialogue with the staff at Helixor, which is prompt, efficient, and usually insightful. Helixor mistletoe, in my experience, gives the strongest fevers and local responses. My clinical results when I switched to only using Helixor mistletoe far surpassed those of any other preparation I used in the past. (All the patients I discussed in chapter 7 were using Helixor mistletoe.)

Unfortunately, Helixor mistletoe is currently available in every country worldwide *except* for the United States. You can fill out an online form and have Helixor mistletoe delivered to your doorstep within weeks if you live in Antarctica, Yemen, Cuba, Haiti, Bolivia, or France, along with explicit directions for use. The only other things you need are a box of 3-ml, ⅝-inch, 25-gauge syringes and a YouTube video on how to give a subcutaneous injection in your abdomen. Delivery and use of these materials are considered safe and legal in every place in the world except the United States. One can only wonder why this is. Again, while it may seem unreasonable to suggest a therapy that is not yet available in the United States, I can only respond that this is a book about my experience with cancer, and my intention is to convey what I have seen works the best.

Limit or Eliminate EMF Exposure

The main premise of this book is that healthy cytoplasmic gel equals good health. When our cytoplasmic gels degrade, our health deteriorates and diseases such as cancer eventually emerge. In the body of the book, I went step by step through the process leading from degradation of the cytoplasmic gels to the eventual emergence of cancer. Cytoplasmic gels are formed from the water in our body, which is then organized into its gel form by the ambient energy sources in our environment. This is shown in one of Dr. Pollack's experiments with the circulation of water in a beaker through hydrophilic tubes. If you place a hydrophilic tube in a beaker of water in a lead box, no gel is formed and there is no flow of water through the tube. But if you take the beaker out of the lead box and shine sunlight on it, a gel layer forms inside the tube. The removal of lead and addition of sunlight separate the charges in the water and the flow begins. The same happens if you place the beaker on the earth or even if you put your hands on the beaker. There are many sources of ambient energy that biological systems can freely use to create gels inside our bodies and cells. This is the energy of life.

One of the main sources (if not *the* main source) of destructive energy that, instead of helping us create healthy gels, degrades our ability to form healthy cytoplasmic gels is in the form of non-ionizing radiation, otherwise known as electromagnetic fields, or EMFs. As long as humans and other life-forms are subject to current levels of non-ionizing radiation, our cancer problem will never be solved. Perhaps the first thing any person with cancer, or any person who suspects she may get cancer, or who is concerned about getting cancer someday (which is all of us), should do is shield herself from EMF exposure to the greatest degree possible.

The scientific research linking EMF exposure from the use of current technologies such as computers, televisions, tablets, cell phones, and all other electronic devices is unequivocal. Normal EMF exposure in the current population is carcinogenic, particularly with the case of brain cancer and even more particularly in the case of brain cancer in children. The relationship is dose dependent, as would be expected from any carcinogenic exposure. That is, the higher the exposure, the more likely it is that cancer will develop. I encourage you to read as much as you can on this subject.[3]

I admittedly have some reluctance in discussing this issue in detail, and part of the reason for that is the sense of futility it engenders. (I also feel there is so much more I need to learn myself, as the subject is vast.) It's not clear that there is any way forward for people to protect themselves from current and normal EMF exposure. Furthermore, with the rollout of 5G beginning in 2019, the situation is likely to get exponentially worse. It is possible that in the next two years, biological life on earth will face a toxic exposure that will make previous encounters with things like plutonium, DDT, and plastics look like child's play. It is not enough for us to claim that because you don't "feel" anything when exposed to EMFs, they can't have an adverse effect. We learned the fallacy of that thinking through our encounter with routine X-rays.

Lately, however, I have learned about strategies that allow individuals to at least lessen some of the damage from EMF exposure. Again, appendix A (page 163) has more information on these strategies. I now urge anyone with cancer to not only consider using these strategies as soon as possible but to actually implement them. As in, right now. While the research on the therapeutic effect of these interventions is currently lacking, they have all been shown to at least reduce the deleterious effects that EMF exposure has on some aspect of our biology. The first are simple bracelets made by Energy Armor, which are impregnated with crystals that seem to reduce the toxic effects of normal and common EMF exposure. These bracelets are best used with grounding and earthing mats, which are sold by Radiant Life.

The second intervention is the sauna therapy within the Faraday cage made by SaunaSpace. Sauna therapy with incandescent and red light therapy has been shown to mitigate some of the effects of EMF exposure, and this product allows your sauna to be done in a "tent" that shields out EMF exposure. And, finally, there are now simple technologies you can use that will turn your bedroom into an EMF-free zone. Doing so allows you to at least spend eight-plus hours per day in an "ancestral" space that contains only the ambient EMF levels (i.e., before humans intervened). The hope is this will allow your body to heal at night, mitigating some of the toxic effects of EMF exposure. Shielded Healing is a company that offers these technologies as well as EMF home assessments.

Information about EMFs belongs in any book concerning human health and disease. Ultimately, we need to come to grips with the fact that we are destroying the possibility for healthy biological life to exist on the earth. No studies have been done to demonstrate the safety of the most massive technological rollout in history. We are in the midst of an existential, spiritual crisis. The resolution of this crisis may determine our future.

Other Interventions

There are, of course, an almost endless number of valuable, nontoxic interventions that have helped and will continue to help people suffering from any number of illnesses, including cancer. The ones I have included are, in my experience, the most promising therapies, and all support my thesis on the etiology of cancer. There are some other interventions that are worth mentioning briefly that can also be supportive.

Sauna Therapy

It should come as no surprise that any therapy that simulates a fever should be helpful for cancer patients. One such ancient therapy is the use of various sauna or heat therapies such as sweat lodges. Sauna therapy that combines the gel "cleansing" effects of sweating with the immune stimulation of heat, along with the energetic boost from the exposure to certain wavelengths of light, fosters our goal of producing healthier intracellular gels. The sauna device meeting these requirements is the SaunaSpace system. This device combines heat and color therapy and does so in a zero-EMF Faraday enclosure. As with any sauna, its use should be individualized, but generally people do about twenty to thirty minutes per day.

Vitamin C

High-dose vitamin C, particularly given intravenously, is another important therapeutic approach for cancer patients. High-dose vitamin C turns into hydrogen peroxide inside the cells, which is highly toxic, specifically to many types of cancer cells. It can be considered a minimally toxic form of chemotherapy. Vitamin C is also a necessary cofactor in the formation of collagen, the proteins that form the intracellular matrix upon which intracellular water is structured. And, finally, vitamin C helps improve immune function, which will be helpful for many people struggling with chronic disease.

While most high-dose vitamin C is given intravenously, in the past few years newer liposomal forms have been shown to produce almost the same effect as IV use. Since cancer cells take up vitamin C, which is chemically similar to glucose, more ardently under fasting conditions, you can safely and effectively give high-dose liposomal vitamin C at the end of a short fast to good effect. I start at hour sixteen of a daily intermittent fast with five grams of oral liposomal vitamin C every fifteen minutes for ten doses. This means an intake of fifty grams of liposomal vitamin C, about the same dose used in most IV therapies. At the end of the ten doses, wait thirty minutes, and then you can break the fast. You can do this two to three times per week for many months to good effect in many cancer cases.

Coffee Enemas

Coffee enemas are a simple, straightforward intervention found in many holistic cancer therapies. The rationale is simple. The rectally infused caffeine dilates the common bile duct, allowing the bile to drain more easily into the small intestine. (This is like being more efficient in taking all of your garbage out to curb, thus preventing the buildup of toxins in your blood, cells, and tissues.) Gerson therapy often includes coffee enemas every two to four hours during the intensive phase. Many people find doing a daily coffee enema to be helpful in improving their overall well-being and preventing the sick and lethargic feeling that comes with being unable to clear out toxins. There are many good directions for coffee enemas on the web, including the best equipment to use, the amount of coffee to use, and even the best source of enema "grade" coffee.

———————

As I pointed out at the beginning of this chapter, all treatment frameworks are by necessity formulaic and therefore limited. However, it is my hope that this framework will stimulate dialogue with your health practitioner and expand your horizons to what is possible. A new day in cancer therapy is coming and coming soon. The days of our only options being to cut, burn, and poison are numbered. The sooner this new day comes the better.

CHAPTER THIRTEEN

Should You Be
Screened for Cancer?

We live in a surveillance state—and this includes medical surveillance. By this I mean we are told (sometimes ordered) to have yearly tests to "screen" for cancer. If we don't, we may be shamed as *bad* or *stupid*, or given the message that if we get sick, then it's pretty much our own fault for not doing what we were supposed to do. But is there any evidence that these unpleasant and copious screenings actually help us live long and better lives?

For this discussion, I am indebted to the brilliant work of a family doctor and epidemiologist from New Hampshire named H. Gilbert Welch, MD, MPH, who wrote the most important book ever written about the science of screening, titled *Should I Be Tested for Cancer?*[1] In it he lays out the argument that while cancer screening is great for medical business interests, it is not so good for the patient.[2]

In order to understand Welch's basic argument, it is important to establish some definitions. When we refer to *screening*, we are only referring to a test done on a healthy person with no signs or symptoms of the disease for which you are testing. In other words, a mammogram done on a healthy fifty-year-old woman with no symptoms is *screening*, whereas a mammogram done on a women with a bloody discharge from her nipple is *diagnostic*—performed in order to determine the cause of the bleeding. A routine PSA, a test to find prostate cancer, performed on a sixty-five-year-old asymptomatic male is screening. The same test performed on a sixty-five-year-old man who is unable to pass urine is diagnostic. In this chapter, I am only discussing screening, not the use of these same tests to find the cause of a particular symptom or group of symptoms.

It seems obvious and hardly even worth discussion that finding cancer early is preferable to finding cancer at a later stage, perhaps when it has already metastasized. It seems so obvious, in fact, that some people even question the need to study the efficacy of cancer screening at all. I myself have said in earlier chapters that stage 4 cancer is very difficult to successfully treat and that it rarely if ever spontaneously resolves on its own. You might think I'd be a most vocal advocate for aggressive cancer screening, if for no other reasons than that finding cancer early would seem to give my holistic therapies a far greater chance of success than treating people whose cancer is further along.

The problem is that when we dig deeper and actually do studies that attempt to show the benefits of screening for cancer, a different, more problematic picture emerges. This picture is further clouded because these days everyone seems to know an "Aunt Bessie who, thank God, caught her breast cancer early, had surgery, radiation, and chemo, and is alive ten years later." How can we not be grateful that she is alive today as a result of our screening programs? Well, we have to turn our attention to the studies on cancer screening to find out what may have really happened to Aunt Bessie.

When we screen for a potentially aggressive disease such as cancer, it is important to realize that "catching it early" may not necessarily lead to a different clinical outcome and that catching the disease earlier makes studying different outcomes particularly problematic. For example, if we are studying a cancer that typically spreads from its original location (the primary site) to distant sites within a year, such as pancreatic cancer, it should be clear that screening for pancreatic cancer every ten years will probably not result in a significant change in outcome. A CT scan of the pancreas every ten years would only show the cancer six months after the prior screening. The following wait of 9.5 more years before the next screening would be too long; the person would be long dead from the pancreatic cancer before the next screening. A patient would have to be extremely lucky for the tumor to show up on the scan in the few months before the ten-year screening in order to truly catch it early on. This is relevant for all screenings. By definition, they will always preferentially catch slower-growing and therefore less aggressive or dangerous cancers. The faster-growing cancers, those that lead to the worst prognosis, are not caught by the screening and are usually found only through the presentation of symptoms.

The natural consequence is that cancer-screening studies will always show higher "cure" rates compared to not screening, while at the same time failing to show overall better outcomes.

We are told that from the time the first breast cancer cell appears to when it can be seen on a screening mammogram is about eight to ten years. By the time the cancer can be felt, it has been present for ten to twelve years. We don't know if catching the cancer two years earlier has any clinical relevance, particularly given the modern treatment for breast cancer. And, as I've tried to make clear in this book, cancer is not the tumor; the tumor is simply a sign that the cancer exists. Cancer is a disease of the cytoplasm and the structuring of water inside the cell. Removing the tumor earlier does not change the course of the disease. As Welch and a colleague concluded in a 2011 paper following a large-scale trial, "Most women with screen-detected breast cancer have not had their life saved by screening. They are instead either diagnosed early (with no effect on their mortality) or overdiagnosed."[3]

In studies, Welch and colleagues found no overall survival benefit from screening for breast cancer with mammograms or screening for ovarian cancer with a CA-125 test.[4] The cure rate goes up for the simple reason that if you remove the breasts of women who have the presence of cancer cells, most will not die of breast cancer. The problem is their overall mortality rate either has no change or in some cases gets a bit worse. In other words, we cured the cancer but the patient dies anyway.

These complexities make statistics on survival duration among patients who undergo screening very difficult to interpret and fraught with the possibility of fraud. For example, if we compare the survival duration of a group of women who discovered breast cancer through mammography screening to those who felt a lump in their breast themselves, we find that the screened women live two years longer on average than the unscreened women. But it should be obvious that the reason is that the survival clock starts two years earlier with screening. If you start the clock two years earlier, it's not really a cause for celebration when people live two years longer.

Two additional studies by Welch demonstrate this with prostate cancer and malignant melanoma of the skin.[5] Dermatologists remove millions of "melanoma" lesions from Americans every year. They, therefore, cure millions of people from deadly melanoma. But as Welch's study shows, the prognosis for melanoma patients has not changed in decades. The same thing applies to men with prostate cancer. We take out millions of prostates with a small amount of cancer each year only to find that if we had done "watchful waiting" (i.e., done nothing), the prognosis is almost identical. Again, "curing" the prostate cancer has no effect on the survival of the patient.

In a similar study, Welch looked at claims that screening for lung cancer with CT scans improved patient prognosis, but found no benefit obtained from this massive screening effort.

"We conclude with 2 fundamental principles that physicians should remember when thinking about screening: (1) survival is always prolonged by early detection, even when deaths are not delayed nor any lives saved, and (2) randomized trials are the only way to reliably determine whether screening does more good than harm."[6]

Perhaps the most shocking result that Welch discovered in his research, and a finding that may explain most of the above lack of benefit from screening tests, is that early, small cancers, the ones most often detected by screening tests, actually can and do remit and go away on their own. A fourteen-year-long breast cancer screening study undertaken by Welch is cloaked in cautious scientific language, but his point is clear: Cancers found by screening exam can and do go away on their own. "Because the cumulative incidence among controls never reached that of the screened group, it appears that some breast cancers detected by repeated mammographic screening would not persist to be detectable by a single mammogram at the end of 6 years. This raises the possibility that the natural course of some screen-detected invasive breast cancers is to spontaneously regress."[7]

Those early cancers we are curing by the millions by catching them on our screening exams? Many of them would have gone away by themselves if we had never bothered to look. Remember Aunt Bessie? If she had never gone for that mammogram, it is possible her early cancer would have remitted on its own, sparing her the trauma, expense, worry, and toxicity of the usual round of surgery, radiation, and toxic chemotherapy. The trouble is that, at this point, we have no idea which cancers will remit on their own and which ones will grow and become a problem. The only area in which this idea has been put into practice even to a small degree is in the treatment of prostate cancer. With prostate cancer, it has been found that watchful waiting is just as effective as an aggressive surgical approach. If that is so, then what is the point of screening besides enriching the people and organizations involved in America's massive cancer care industry?

Over the years, many people have tried to interest me in various techniques and strategies for early cancer detection in my patients. These include thermography, blood tests such as the AMSA test, and even the sensitive crystallization used in some anthroposophical clinics. While these and many more tests may be helpful in finding some cancers and may also be helpful in following the progress of cancer treatments, when it comes to screening large segments of the population, I have to agree with Welch that until we see clear randomized trials that show an improvement in overall health outcomes as a result of screening, I simply can't get behind screening tests.

I started this chapter by pointing out the insidious nature of life in a surveillance society. The examples I cover are a minuscule fraction of the surveillance and intrusion into our privacy, including our medical privacy, that we are subjected to on a routine basis and have become, I fear, desensitized to. I am simply not willing to condone regular surveillance of our bodies without evidence that it provides any benefit to our health. At this point, I don't believe that evidence exists.

My suspicion is that the whole concept of screening is flawed. I understand this means that people would be living with more uncertainty and would be in conflict with their usual health care providers. I understand that it is considered heretical to not subject yourself to periodic investigation on the status of your health. But I also think we need to consider the repercussions to our sense of freedom and integrity that this scrutiny entails, and an overall sense of living in a constant state of fear that it engenders. Fundamentally, I at least want people to clearly understand the issues involved and, without any coercion of any sort, each to feel free to choose her own course of action. To my mind, that would be the best outcome from raising this difficult subject and the reason why I'm doing it.

Marcia Angell, MD, former executive editor of the *New England Journal of Medicine*, arguably the most prestigious medical journal in the world, made a statement in 2009 that gets to the core of the issues we are facing: "It is simply no longer possible to believe much of the clinical research that is published, or to rely on the judgment of trusted physicians or authoritative medical guidelines. I take no pleasure in this conclusion, which I reached slowly and reluctantly over my two decades as an editor of *The New England Journal of Medicine*."

Conclusion

We live our lives based on the stories we tell ourselves. Cultures are defined by the stories we tell each other. If we want to change what is happening in our lives or in our culture, we must change the story. Right now, if you'll permit an allegory, we are living out the story of *Sleeping Beauty*. The kingdom, which represents the condition of peace and justice, is under the spell of an evil, scorned witch—the symbol of materialistic thinking and the belief that only material substance exists.

This depiction is mirrored by the description of reality we find in quantum physics. The manifest, physical world can exist in at least two distinct states. One is as a particle; the other is as a wave. When matter exists as particles, it represents the material nature of atoms. When atoms exist as a wave, they are more fluid, less material, acting as energy. Physicists say that what determines whether any atom will show up as a particle or a wave depends on whether it is being observed. In other words, the actual, literal state of the building blocks of matter is determined by the conscious observer. Some physicists even go so far as to say consciousness "dreamed" the physical world into existence.

In *Sleeping Beauty*, the princess, who represents the salvation of the kingdom, a state of harmony, peace, health, and the

159

maternal, watery cytoplasm consciousness, is asleep. She is under the spell of the materialistic, particle-bound, nucleus-like consciousness of the evil witch. The fate of the kingdom depends on whether the princess will awaken from the spell and recognize herself for who she truly is. That is, she must awaken and see the world of matter as a kind of spell into which we unwittingly fall. She must awaken from this spell, not to a new world, but to awareness of her true nature.

Our current culture—and nowhere can this be seen more clearly than in medicine and oncology—is suffering under the same spell. We have been bewitched by the promises of materialism and the "particle" way of seeing the world. Under this spell, we have built great buildings, dams, and structures. We have explored the heavens and the depths of the seas. We have built great computers capable of doing almost unimaginable things. We have decided that the human being consists only of material substance and functions much like a machine. And we have decided that the cause of cancer is oncogenes, rather than the life forces that reside in the watery cytoplasm. As a result, we are not only asleep to our true nature; we are doomed. People and cultures that only see, only acknowledge, the material nature of life are not only seeing the world incorrectly, but inevitably destroy the life of the only home they have. They attempt to turn life into money and in turn destroy the living earth. This is the story of our culture and of the disease called cancer.

The way out of this tragic situation is also shown to us in *Sleeping Beauty*. The princess can wake up, the kingdom can become a place of peace, abundance, and harmony, but only through the intervention of the "handsome prince." The prince brings the simplest, most profound gift of all to the princess and to all of humanity. It is the gift of love. Love is the force, the energy, the power in the world that can awaken us from this deep slumber. Love, whether between people, toward animals, or toward the entire miracle of creation, awakens us to the reality of who we truly are. In *Sleeping Beauty*, it is through love, the kiss of the prince, that the princess awakens to her true nature. She can finally see herself as a spiritual being in human form: a being who can reside in both worlds and create a harmony of the two. This is the story of the yin-yang symbol and the story of the birth of Jesus. It is the story of the dense, physical nucleus with the watery, living cytoplasm. It is the story of cancer and the challenge for our culture. Either we can wake up to our true nature, and soon, or we are destined to destroy everything. Which will you choose?

Recommended Sources of Therapies and Medicines

The choice of where to get the products and medicines I recommend throughout this book is usually pretty straightforward. In all cases, I considered as many aspects of how the final product was obtained as possible. This included where the food or plant was grown, and how it is processed, stored, and distributed. In some cases, I chose a company because the founder has dedicated a good portion of his or her career to studying the product in question, such as Dr. George Birkmayer's NADH.

There have been instances when I was unable to find reliable sources of a certain plant or medicine, so one of my two family businesses (Dr. Cowan's Garden and Human Heart, Cosmic Heart) has made it available. This is the case with ashitaba and our *Strophanthus* capsules. I realize this may seem self-serving, but in both cases our family business was the only avenue for bringing a totally biodynamically grown or wild-harvested, correctly processed product to market. It's been a case of "if you want something done right, you have to do it yourself." With that introduction, here is the list of where to obtain the products I mention in chapter 12.

Ashitaba. As far as we know, Dr. Cowan's Garden (www
.drcowansgarden.com) provides the only domestically produced ashitaba product available. Our ashitaba is obtained
from two stellar biodynamic growers in Northern California, who dry it and ship it to be ground and packed at our
kitchen in West Virginia.

Burdock root. Right now there is only one commercial organic
burdock grower of any consequence in the United States.
Its product is available through Dr. Cowan's Garden (www
.drcowansgarden.com). We obtain our burdock root
directly from this source, dry it, and grind it into an easy-
to-use powder, stored in our Miron jars.

Chaga tea. There are now many good sources of wildcrafted
chaga products available on the internet. You can source a
wildcrafted tincture through Raw Revelations (www.raw
revelations.com) and though Human Heart, Cosmic Heart
(www.humanheartcosmicheart.com).

Deuterium-depleted water. Currently I know of two companies that are selling DDW in the United States. The Center
for Deuterium Depletion (www.ddcenters.com) carries different strengths of DDW and makes these available to its
clients. Divinia (www.diviniawater.com) sells water that has
a slightly lower deuterium content than most commercially
sold waters, but it's not low enough to be of value in
treatment.

EMF bracelets and grounding mats. Energy Armor (www
.energy-armor.com) carries several bracelets that reduce the
toxic effects of EMF exposure. Grounding and earthing
mats can be purchased through the Radiant Life catalog
(www.radiantlifecatalog.com).

EMF home assessments and solutions. Shielded Healing
offers home assessments and recommends a variety of products that can help mitigate EMF exposure in your home.
You can book assessments and consultations, purchase

products, and learn more about EMF exposure on its website (shieldedhealing.com).

Food. The only thing that needs mentioning here is the Weston A. Price Foundation shopping guide can be an invaluable resource in obtaining the best-quality foods. It is especially helpful in obtaining harder-to-find items like bone broth and naturally fermented vegetables.

Liposomal vitamin C. There are many good brands of liposomal vitamin C. I prefer non-GMO, noncorn versions, such as the one we carry through Human Heart, Cosmic Heart (www.humanheartcosmicheart.com). Quicksilver Scientific (www.quicksilverscientific.com) also carries a premium form of liposomal vitamin C.

Mistletoe. The best source of mistletoe is through Helixor's website (www.helixor.com). Through the website, the staff at Helixor also offer recommendations on the preparation best suited to your individual case along with the dosing instructions. As I noted in chapter 12, the United States is currently the only country in the world where Helixor mistletoe cannot legally be shipped, but hopefully this situation will change in the near future. Currently there are very few other avenues to obtain mistletoe ampules in the United States.

NADH. The important thing to know about NADH is the Birkmayer Rapid Energy packets are the only ones that have produced consistent results. I obtain them directly from Prof. George Birkmayer NADH (www.birkmayer-nadh .com). They are also available from Human Heart, Cosmic Heart (www.humanheartcosmicheart.com).

Quinton isotonic seawater. You can get this in either individual-serving foil packets or in one-liter glass bottles. I prefer the glass bottles, but as of this writing they are not available on the internet. This may change soon, but in the meantime you can obtain the packets either from Quicksilver

Scientific (www.quicksilverscientific.com) or from Human
Heart, Cosmic Heart (www.humanheartcosmicheart.com).

Sauna. The best sauna comes from SaunaSpace (www.sauna
space.com). If possible, it is best used inside the company's
patented Faraday cage, which shields out incoming EMF
interferences.

***Strophanthus* capsules.** Human Heart, Cosmic Heart (www
.humanheartcosmicheart.com) offers the only pure
Strophanthus seed capsules available in the United States.
Our seeds are harvested from 300 to 400 foot vines in
Cameroon by members of the Baka tribe who have harvested *Strophanthus* for centuries. The seeds are collected,
dried, sent to Germany for processing, and then distributed
in the United States through Human Heart, Cosmic Heart.

Turmeric. The best-quality ground turmeric can be obtained
from either Burlap & Barrel (www.burlapandbarrel.com) or
from Dr. Cowan's Garden (www.drcowansgarden.com).

APPENDIX B

The Physiological Significance of St. George Slaying the Dragon and *The Birth of Venus*

I f you examine various paintings of St. George and the dragon by Renaissance masters such as van Dyck and Raphael, you often see St. George atop a white stallion brandishing a red sword in his right arm. It often appears as if the sword is emerging from the right upper quadrant of the abdomen, known as McBurney's point, where gall bladder pain is typically felt. In fact, when a technician performs an ultrasound exam of a patient's abdomen for gall bladder disease, he will typically report the patient's pain, or lack of pain, when pressing the ultrasound wand right over McBurney's point. In esoteric lore, the dragon is associated with the sulfurous, unconscious processes that occur in the metabolic region, below the diaphragm. Human evolution is intimately linked with the development of consciousness, and St. George is one of the mythical figures guiding humanity in that development. He is the messenger from Mars, the red planet; in esoteric traditions the gall bladder is the organ associated with Mars and the metal iron.

So what van Dyck and Raphael are demonstrating is that St. George works through our gall bladder to bring iron into our being. The function of iron is to detoxify, and by combining with the heme molecule, St. George slays the sulfurous, unconscious impulses that lie in our metabolic realm. By slaying the dragon, we become more awake, conscious beings able to co-create a universe that can work for everyone. When we succumb to our unconscious impulses, we risk becoming tools for death and destruction.

In Botticelli's *The Birth of Venus*, we see an azure blue painting that depicts the goddess Venus, also known as Aphrodite, emerging from the sea, riding on an open clamshell. Venus, the goddess, is said to be the representative of the planet Venus on earth and the goddess of love and sensuality. In esoteric lore, Venus, both the planet and the goddess, is connected to copper and to the kidneys. Clam blood, in fact, is copper-based, not iron-based like mammal blood, and due to this copper base, it is the shade of azure blue depicted in the painting, rather than red like the blood of mammals. The painting evokes strong sensual imagery as if to remind us that the sensual, emotional world is based on the element of copper and associated with the kidneys. While this may seem strange to modern physiologists, we now know that the hat that sits on top of our kidneys, called the adrenal gland, plays a large role in our emotional and sexual well-being. Botticelli is reminding us of the physiological role of copper in this dramatic rendition of the goddess of love and emotions emerging out of the copper realm. In some analyses of this painting, we are told that Venus alights in our world on the ancient island of Crete, a place that, not coincidentally, has some of the world's richest copper deposits.

NOTES

Foreword

1. Lisa Rapaport, "U.S. Health Spending Twice Other Countries' with Worse Results," *Reuters Health News*, March 13, 2018, https://www.reuters.com/article/us-health-spending/u-s-health-spending-twice-other-countries-with-worse-results-idUSKCN1GP2YN.

Introduction

1. Ulrich R. Abel, "Chemotherapy of Advanced Epithelial Cancer—A Critical Review," *Biomedicine and Pharmacotherapy* 46, no. 10 (1992): 439–52, https://doi.org/10.1016/0753-3322(92)90002-O.
2. Abel, "Chemotherapy of Advanced Epithelial Cancer."
3. Abel, "Chemotherapy of Advanced Epithelial Cancer."
4. Ulrich R. Abel, *Cytostatic Chemotherapy of Advanced Epithelial Tumors: A Critical Inventory* (Stuttgart, Germany: Hippokrates Verlag, 1995).
5. G. Morgan, R. Ward, and M. Barton, "The Contribution of Cytotoxic Chemotherapy to 5-Year Survival in Adult Malignancies," abstract, *Clinical Oncology* 16, no. 8 (December 2004), https://www.ncbi.nlm.nih.gov/pubmed/15630849?report=abstract.
6. Sylvie Beljanski, "Are We Winning the War on Cancer? The Good News," *Newsweek*, February 25, 2019, https://www.newsweek.com/are-we-winning-war-cancer-good-news-799096.

7. "Our Research Programs," American Cancer Society, accessed February 25, 2019, https://www.cancer.org/research.html.

8. American Cancer Society, "Cancer Deaths Drop for Second Consecutive Year," *Science News, ScienceDaily*, accessed February 25, 2019, https://www.sciencedaily.com/releases /2007/01/070118095233.htm.

9. American Cancer Society, "Cancer Deaths Drop."

10. Clifton Leaf, "Why We're Losing the War on Cancer (and How to Win It)," *Fortune*, March 22, 2004, http://fortune .com/2004/03/22/cancer-medicines-drugs-health/.

Chapter 1: The Failure of the Oncogene Theory

1. Ulrich Pfeffer, ed., *Cancer Genomics: Molecular Classification, Prognosis and Response Prediction* (Dordrecht, Netherlands: Springer Science+Business Media, 2013), 47, https://doi .org/10.1007/978-94-007-5842-1_2.

2. Sebastian Salas-Vega, Othon Iliopoulos, and Elias Mossialos, "Assessment of Overall Survival, Quality of Life, and Safety Benefits Associated with New Cancer Medicines," *JAMA Oncology* 3, no. 3 (2017): 382–90, https://doi.org/10.1001 /jamaoncol.2016.4166.

3. Salas-Vega et al., "Assessment of Overall Survival."

4. Courtney Davis et al., "Availability of Evidence of Benefits on Overall Survival and Quality of Life of Cancer Drugs Approved by European Medicines Agency: Retrospective Cohort Study of Drug Approvals 2009–13," *British Medical Journal*, no. 4530 (October 4, 2017): 359, https:// doi.org/10.1136/bmj.j4530.

5. Davis et al., "Availability of Evidence."

6. Davis et al., "Availability of Evidence."

7. Ellen R. Copson et al., "Germline BRCA Mutation and Outcome in Young-Onset Breast Cancer (POSH): A Prospective Cohort Study," *Lancet Oncology* 19, no. 2 (February 1, 2018): 169–80, https://doi.org/10.1016 /S1470-2045(17)30891-4.

8. Copson et al., "Germline BRCA Mutation."
9. Cheryl Lin et al., "The Case against BRCA 1 and 2 Testing," *Surgery* 149, no. 6 (June 2011): 731–34, https://doi.org/10.1016/j.surg.2010.11.009.
10. Alexandra J. Van den Broek et al., "Worse Breast Cancer Prognosis of BRCA1/BRCA2 Mutation Carriers: What's the Evidence? A Systematic Review with Meta-Analysis," *PLOS ONE* 10, no. 3 (March 27, 2015), http://doi.org/10.1371/journal.pone.0120189.
11. Leslie A. Pray, "Gleevec: The Breakthrough in Cancer Treatment," *Nature Education* 1, no.1 (2008): 37, https://www.nature.com/scitable/topicpage/gleevec-the-breakthrough-in-cancer-treatment-565.

Chapter 2: The Locus of Cancer

1. Thomas N. Seyfried, *Cancer as a Metabolic Disease: On the Origin, Management and Prevention of Cancer* (Hoboken, NJ: John Wiley and Sons, 2012): 195–206.
2. See my previous book, *Vaccines, Autoimmunity, and the Changing Nature of Childhood Illness* (White River Junction, VT: Chelsea Green Publishing, 2018), for a full discussion.

Chapter 3: What Is Life?

1. Erwin Schrödinger, *What Is Life? The Physical Aspect of the Living Cell* (Cambridge, UK: Cambridge University Press, 1944).
2. See my previous book, *Vaccines, Autoimmunity, and the Changing Nature of Childhood Illness*, for a full discussion.

Chapter 4: Quinton Isotonic Plasma

1. Laboratoires Quinton, *Special Report: Seawater*, 2018, http://quinton.no/wp-content/uploads/2018/06/INFORME_ESPECIAL_ingles.pdf.
2. Laboratoires Quinton, *Special Report: Seawater*.
3. Laboratoires Quinton, *Special Report: Seawater*.

4. Laboratoires Quinton, *Special Report: Seawater*.
5. Hee Sun Hwang et al., "Anti-Obesity and Antidiabetic Effects of Deep Sea Water on *ob/ob* Mice," *Marine Biotechnology* 11, no. 4 (July 2009): 531.
6. Hwang et al., "Anti-Obesity and Antidiabetic Effects of Deep Sea Water."
7. Geethalakshmi Radhakrishnan et al., "Intake of Dissolved Organic Matter from Deep Seawater Inhibits Atherosclerosis Progression," *Biochemical and Biophysical Research Communications* 387, no. 1 (September 11, 2009): 25–30, https://doi.org/10.1016/j.bbrc.2009.06.073.
8. Saburo Yoshioka et al., "Pharmacological Activity of Deep-Sea Water: Examination of Hyperlipemia Prevention and Medical Treatment Effect," *Biological and Pharmaceutical Bulletin* 26, no. 11 (December 2003): 1552–9, https://doi.org/10.1248/bpb.26.1552.
9. H. Kimata, H. Tai, and H. Nakajima, "Reduction of Allergic Skin Responses and Serum Allergen-Specific IgE and IgE-Inducing Cytokines by Drinking Deep-Sea Water in Patients with Allergic Rhinitis," *Otorhinolaryngologia Nova* 11 (2001): 302–3, https://doi.org/10.1159/000068306.

Chapter 5: Gerson Therapy

1. I discuss this at length in my previous book, *Vaccines, Autoimmunity, and the Changing Nature of Childhood Illness*.
2. F. W. Cope, "A Medical Application of the Ling Association-Induction Hypothesis: The High Potassium, Low Sodium Diet of the Gerson Cancer Therapy," *Physiological Chemistry and Physics* 10, no. 5 (1978): 465–8, https://www.ncbi.nlm.nih.gov/pubmed/751080.
3. G. L. Gar Hildenbrand et al., "Five-Year Survival Rates of Melanoma Patients Treated by Diet Therapy after the Manner of Gerson: A Retrospective Review," *Alternative Therapies in Health and Medicine* 1, no. 4 (1995): 29–37, https://pdfs.semanticscholar.org/91fc/8294810a11e7e70b

9fee3cb89d4b29678ffa.pdf; Max Gerson, "The Cure of Advanced Cancer by Diet Therapy: A Summary of 30 Years of Clinical Experimentation," *Physiological Chemistry and Physics* 10, no. 5 (1978): 449–64, https://www.ncbi.nlm.nih .gov/pubmed/751079.

Chapter 6: Cardiac Glycosides

1. B. Stenkvist, "Is Digitalis a Therapy for Breast Carcinoma?" *Oncology Reports* 6, no. 3 (May 1999): 493–9, https://doi .org/10.3892/or.6.3.493.

2. J. Haux, "Digitoxin Is a Potential Anticancer Agent for Several Types of Cancer," *Medical Hypotheses* 53, no. 6 (December 1999): 543–8, https://doi.org/10.1054/mehy .1999.0985.

3. M. Iltaf Khan, "Digitalis, a Targeted Therapy for Cancer?" *American Journal of the Medical Sciences* 337, no. 5 (May 2009): 355–9, https://doi.org/10.1097/MAJ.0b013e318 1942f57.

4. Jin-Qiang Chen et al., "Sodium/Potassium ATPase (Na+, K+-ATPase) and Ouabain/Related Cardiac Glycosides: A New Paradigm for Development of Anti-Breast Cancer Drugs?" *Breast Cancer Research and Treatment* 96, no. 1 (March 2006): 1–15, https://doi.org/10.1007/s10549 -005-9053-3.

5. See my book *Human Heart, Cosmic Heart : A Doctor's Quest to Understand, Treat, and Prevent Cardiovascular Disease* (White River Junction, VT: Chelsea Green Publishing, 2016).

6. Yung-Luen Shih et al., "Ouabain Impairs Cell Migration and Invasion and Alters Gene Expression of Human Osteosarcoma U-2 OS Cells," *Environmental Toxicology* 32, no. 11 (November 2017): 2400–13, https://doi.org/10.1002/tox.22453; Thidarat Ruanghirun, Varisa Pongrakhananon, and Pithi Chanvorachote, "Ouabain Enhances Lung Cancer Cell Detachment," *Anticancer Research* 34, no. 5 (May 2014): 2231–8, http://ar.iiarjournals

.org/content/34/5/2231.full; Yijun Xiao et al., "Ouabain Targets the Na/K-ATPase a3 to Inhibit Cancer Cell Proliferation and Induce Apoptosis," *Oncology Letters* 14, no. 6 (December 2017): 6678–84, http://doi.org/10.3892/ol.2017.7070.

Chapter 7: Plant and Mushroom Medicines

1. C. Louis Kervran, *Biological Transmutations*, trans. Michel Abehsera (Magalia, CA: Happiness Press, 1989).

2. Hae Min So et al., "Bioactivity Evaluations of Betulin Identified from the Bark of *Betula platyphylla* var. *japonica* for Cancer Therapy," *Archives of Pharmacal Research* 41, no. 8 (August 2018): 815–22, https://doi.org/10.1007/s12272-018-1064-9.

3. Antoine Géry et al., "Chaga (*Inonotus obliquus*), a Future Potential Medicinal Fungus in Oncology? A Chemical Study and a Comparison of the Cytotoxicity against Human Lung Adenocarcinoma Cells (A549) and Human Bronchial Epithelial Cells (BEAS-2B)," *Integrative Cancer Therapies* 17, no. 3 (September 2018): 832–43, http://doi.org/10.1177/1534735418757912.

4. Yusuke Baba et al., "Arctigenin Induces the Apoptosis of Primary Effusion Lymphoma Cells under Conditions of Glucose Starvation," *International Journal of Oncology* 52, no. 2 (February 2018): 505–17, https://doi.org/10.3892/ijo.2017.4215.

5. Piwen Wang et al., "Increased Chemopreventive Effect by Combining Arctigenin, Green Tea Polyphenol and Curcumin in Prostate and Breast Cancer Cells," *RSC Advances* 4, no. 66 (August 2014): 35242–50, http://doi.org/10.1039/C4RA06616B.

6. Yinghua He et al., "Molecular Mechanisms of the Action of Arctigenin in Cancer," *Biomedicine and Pharmacotherapy* 108 (December 2018): 403–7, https://doi.org/10.1016/j.biopha.2018.08.158.

7. En-Hui Zhang et al., "An Update on Antitumor Activity of Naturally Occurring Chalcones," *Evidence-Based Complementary and Alternative Medicine* 2013, Article ID 815621 (April 2013), http://doi.org/10.1155/2013/815621.

8. Florian Pelzer, "Complementary Treatment with Mistletoe Extracts during Chemotherapy: Safety, Neutropenia, Fever, and Quality of Life Assessed in a Randomized Study," *Journal of Alternative and Complementary Medicine* 24 (September 2018): 954–61, http://doi.org/10.1089/acm.2018.0159.

9. Tycho Jan Zuzak et al., "Safety of High-Dose Intravenous Mistletoe Therapy in Pediatric Cancer Patients: A Case Series," *Complementary Therapies in Medicine* 40 (October 2018): 198–202, https://doi.org/10.1016/j.ctim.2018.01.002.

10. Yun-Gyoo Lee et al., "Efficacy and Safety of *Viscum album* Extract (Helixor-M) to Treat Malignant Pleural Effusion in Patients with Lung Cancer," *Supportive Care in Cancer* (2018): 1–5, https://doi.org/10.1007/s00520-018-4455-z.

11. Friedemann Schad et al., "Overall Survival of Stage IV Non-Small Cell Lung Cancer Patients Treated with *Viscum album* L. in Addition to Chemotherapy, a Real-World Observational Multicenter Analysis," *PLOS ONE* 13, no. 8 (August 2018), https://doi.org/10.1371/journal.pone.0203058.

12. Jan Axtner et al., "Health Services Research of Integrative Oncology in Palliative Care of Patients with Advanced Pancreatic Cancer," *BMC Cancer* 16 (August 2016), https://doi.org/10.1186/s12885-016-2594-5.

13. Johannes Gutsch et al., "Complete Remission and Long-Term Survival of a Patient with a Diffuse Large B-Cell Lymphoma under *Viscum album* Extracts after Resistance to R-CHOP: A Case Report," *Anticancer Research* 38, no. 9 (September 2018): 5363–9, http;//doi.org/10.21873/anticanres.12865.

14. Paul Georg Werthmann, Roman Huber, and Gunver Sophia Kienle, "Durable Clinical Remission of a Skull Metastasis under Intralesional Viscum album Extract Therapy: Case Report," *Head and Neck* 40, no. 7 (July 2018): E77–E81, https://doi.org/10.1002/hed.25320.
15. Achim Rose et al., "Mistletoe Plant Extract in Patients with Nonmuscle Invasive Bladder Cancer: Results of a Phase Ib/IIa Single Group Dose Escalation Study," *The Journal of Urology* 4 (October 2015): 939–43, https://doi.org/10.1016/j.juro.2015.04.073.
16. Maurice Orange, Uwe Reuter, and Uwe Hobohm, "Coley's Lessons Remembered: Augmenting Mistletoe Therapy," *Integrative Cancer Therapies* 15, no. 4 (December 2016): 502–11, http://doi.org/10.1177/1534735416649916.

Chapter 8: The Ketogenic Diet

1. Vilhjalmur Sefansson, *Cancer: Disease of Civilization? An Anthropological and Historical Study* (New York: Hill and Wang, 1960); Weston A. Price, *Nutrition and Physical Degeneration*, 8th ed. (Lemon Grove, CA: Price-Pottenger Nutrition Foundation, 2009).
2. László G. Boros et al., "Submolecular Regulation of Cell Transformation by Deuterium Depleting Water Exchange Reactions in the Tricarboxylic Acid Substrate Cycle," *Medical Hypotheses* 87 (February 2016): 69–74, https://doi.org/10.1016/j.mehy.2015.11.016.

Chapter 9: Deuterium-Depleted Water

1. Sanctuaires Notre-Dame de Lourdes, *Bilan 2008 et Perspectives 2009* (Lourdes: Service Communication, 2009), 12–22.
2. Bernard François, Esther M. Sternberg, and Elizabeth Fee, "The Lourdes Medical Cures Revisited," *Journal of the History of Medicine and Allied Sciences* 69, no. 1 (July 2012): 135–62, http://doi.org/10.1093/jhmas/jrs041.

3. A. V. Syroeshkin et al., "The Effect of the Deuterium Depleted Water on the Biological Activity of the Eukaryotic Cells," *Journal of Trace Elements in Medicine and Biology* 50 (December 2018): 629–33, https://doi.org/10.1016/j.jtemb.2018.05.004.

4. Syroeshkin et al., "The Effect of the Deuterium Depleted Water."

5. Krisztina Krempels et al., "A Retrospective Study of Survival in Breast Cancer Patients Undergoing Deuterium Depletion in Addition to Conventional Therapies," *Journal of Cancer Research and Therapy* 1, no. 8 (2013): 194–200, http://dx.doi.org/10.14312/2052-4994.2013-29.

6. Krempels et al., "A Retrospective Study."

7. Krempels et al., "A Retrospective Study."

8. András Kovács et al., "Deuterium Depletion May Delay the Progression of Prostate Cancer," *Journal of Cancer Therapy* 2 (2011): 548–56, http://doi.org/10.4236/jct.2011.24075.

9. Kovács et al., "Deuterium Depletion," 555.

10. Krisztina Krempels, Ildikó Somlyai, and Gábor Somlyai, "A Retrospective Evaluation of the Effects of Deuterium Depleted Water Consumption on 4 Patients with Brain Metastases from Lung Cancer," *Integrative Cancer Therapies* 7, no. 3 (September 2018): 172–81, http://doi.org/10.1177/1534735408322851.

Chapter 10: NADH

1. George D. Birkmayer and Jiren Zhang, "NADH in Cancer Prevention and Therapy," in *Phytopharmaceuticals in Cancer Chemoprevention*, ed. Dabasis Bagchi and Harry G. Preuss (Boca Raton, FL: CRC Press, 2004), 541–54.

2. Amanda Garrido and Nabil Djouder, "NAD+ Deficits in Age-Related Diseases and Cancer," *Trends in Cancer* 3, no. 8 (August 2017): 593–l610, http://doi.org/10.1016/j.trecan.2017.06.001; Shunqin Zhu et al., "The Role of Sirtuins Family in Cell Metabolism during Tumor Development," *Seminars in*

Cancer Biology (November 2018), https://doi.org/10.1016/j
.semcancer.2018.11.003; Liang Shi et al., "SIRT5-Mediated
Deacetylation of LDHB Promotes Autophagy and
Tumorigensis in Colorectal Cancer," *Molecular Oncology* 13,
no. 2 (February 2019): 358–75, https://doi.org/10.1002
/1878-0261.12408; Sara Iachettini et al., "Pharmacological
Activation of SIRT6 Triggers Lethal Autophagy in Human
Cancer Cells," *Cell Death and Disease* 9, article no. 996 (2018),
http://doi.org/10.1038 s41419-018-1065-0.

Chapter 11: Energetic Life Forces

1. "Dr. Arthur W. Yale M.D. Talks about Using the Rife
   Machine on His Patients," RifeVideos.com, http://www
   .rifevideos.com/dr_arthur_w_yale_md_talks_about
   _using_the_rife_machine_on_his_patients.html.
2. Barry Lynes, *The Cancer Cure That Worked! Fifty Years of
   Suppression* (S. Lake Tahoe, CA: BioMed Publishing
   Group, 1987), 62.
3. Barry Lynes, *Rife's World of Electromedicine: The Story, the
   Corruption and the Promise* (S. Lake Tahoe, CA: BioMed
   Publishing Group, 2009), 41.
4. Lynes, *Rife's World of Electromedicine*, 51.
5. Jim B. Tucker, *Return to Life: Extraordinary Cases of Children
   Who Remember Past Lives* (New York: St. Martin's Press,
   2013), 167.
6. Tucker, *Return to Life*, 168.
7. Tucker, *Return to Life*, 189.
8. Stephan A. Schwartz and Larry Dossey, "Nonlocality,
   Intention, and Observer Effects in Healing Studies: Laying a
   Foundation for the Future," *Explore* 6, no. 5 (September–
   October 2010): 295–307, http://doi.org/10.1016/j.explore
   .2010.06.011.
9. Cynthia Bourgeault, *The Heart of Centering Prayer: Nondual
   Christianity in Theory and Practice* (Boulder, CO:
   Shambhala, 2016).

Chapter 12: A Basic Cancer Therapy Framework

1. Frank Shallenberger, "Melatonin Isn't Just for Sleeping—
From Cardiovascular Disease and Cancer to Aging and
Macular Degeneration the Research Will Shock You,"
Townsend Letter, February/March 2019.
2. Venkataramanujam Srinivasan, Mahaneem Mohamed, and
Hisanori Kato, "Melatonin in Bacterial and Viral Infections
with Focus on Sepsis: A Review," *Recent Patents on
Endocrine, Metabolic and Immune Drug Discovery* 6, no. 1
(2012): 30–9, doi:10.2174/187221412799015317; Frank
A. J. L. Scheer et al., "Daily Nighttime Melatonin Reduces
Blood Pressure in Male Patients with Essential
Hypertension," *Hypertension* 43 (2004): 192–7, https://
doi.org/10.1161/01.HYP.0000113293.15186.3b; Anna
Gry Vinther and Mogens Helweg Claësson, "The Influence
of Melatonin on the Immune System and Cancer," *Ugeskr
Laeger* 177, no. 21 (May 2015), https://www.ncbi.nlm.nih.
gov/pubmed/26027592; Amit Naskar et al., "Melatonin
Enhances L-Dopa Therapeutic Effects, Helps to Reduce Its
Dose, and Protects Dopaminergic Neurons in 1-methyl-4-
phenyl-1,2,3,6-tetrahydropyridine-Induced Parkinsonism
in Mice," *Journal of Pineal Research* 58, no. 3 (April 2015):
262–74, https://doi.org/10.1111/jpi.12212; Golmaryam
Sarlak et al., "Effects of Melatonin on Nervous System
Again: Neurogenesis and Neurodegeneration," *Journal of
Pharmacological Sciences* 123, no. 1 (August 2013): 9–24,
http://doi.org/10.1254/jphs.13R01SR; N. A. Stefanova et
al., "Potential of Melatonin for Prevention of Age-Related
Macular Degeneration: Experimental Study," *Advances in
Gerontology* 3, no. 4 (October 2013): 302–8, https://doi
.org/10.1134/S2079057013040073; P. Lissoni et al.,
"Decreased Toxicity and Increased Efficacy of Cancer
Chemotherapy Using the Pineal Hormone Melatonin in
Metastatic Solid Tumour Patients with Poor Clinical
Status," *European Journal of Cancer* 35, no. 12 (November

1999): 1688–92, https://doi.org/10.1016/S0959
-8049(99)00159-8; Rosa M. Sainz et al., "Melatonin
Reduces Prostate Cancer Cell Growth Leading to
Neuroendocrine Differentiation via a Receptor and PKA
Independent Mechanism," *The Prostate* 63, no. 1 (April
2005): 29–43, https://doi.org/10.1002/pros.20155;
Edward Mills et al., "Melatonin in the Treatment of
Cancer: A Systematic Review of Randomized Controlled
Trials and Meta-Analysis," *Journal of Pineal Research* 39,
no. 4 (November 2005): 360–6, https://doi.org/10.1111
/j.1600-079X.2005.00258.x.

3. To start, you might read the Children's Health Defense's
article, "The Dangers of 5G to Children's Health" at www
.childrenshealthdefense.org; listen to interviews given by
Dr. Martin Pall, PhD, on the dangers of EMF exposure,
such as this interview on KPFA: http://www.yourown
healthandfitness.org/?page_id=509; and listen to the
lecture given by the well-known Swedish scientist Olle
Johansson, "Electromagnetic Fields and Their Side Effects
on Our Health" at www.emfcommunity.com.

Chapter 13: Should You Be Screened for Cancer?

1. H. Gilbert Welch, *Should I Be Tested for Cancer? Maybe
Not and Here's Why* (Berkeley: University of California
Press, 2006).

2. A 2018 investigation by Dartmouth College, where Welch was
a faculty member, accused him of plagiarizing a graph
published in a 2016 *New England Journal of Medicine* paper,
leading to his resignation, although Welch disputed the
accusations and the *New England Journal of Medicine*
determined there were not "sufficient grounds" to merit
retraction. If you read between the lines, it looks a lot like a
hit job, perhaps due to the nature of Welch's research and the
degree to which it challenges medical private interests, but I
don't know. What I can say is that, in my opinion, the

college's accusations do not detract from the importance of Welch's books or the significance of his work overall, which I feel is of vital importance. It saddens and troubles me that we no longer have his contributions because of a questionable dispute over a graph.

3. H. Gilbert Welch and Brittney A. Frankel, "Likelihood That a Woman with Screen-Detected Breast Cancer Has Had Her 'Life Saved' by That Screening," *Archives of Internal Medicine* 171, no. 22 (2011): 2043–6, http://doi.org /10.1001/archinternmed.2011.476.

4. H. Gilbert Welch and Honor J. Passow, "Quantifying the Benefits and Harms of Screening Mammography," *JAMA Internal Medicine* 174, no. 3 (2014): 448–54, http://doi .org/10.1001/jamainternmed.2013.13635; Archie Bleyer and H. Gilbert Welch, "Effect of Three Decades of Screening Mammography on Breast-Cancer Incidence," *New England Journal of Medicine* 367 (November 2012): 1998–2005, http://doi.org/10.1056/NEJMoa1206809; Saundra S. Buys et al., "Effect of Screening on Ovarian Cancer Mortality: The Prostate, Lung, Colorectal and Ovarian (PLCO) Cancer Screening Randomized Controlled Trial," *JAMA* 305, no. 22 (2011): 2295–2303, http://doi.org/10.1001/jama.2011.766.

5. H. Gilbert Welch and Peter C. Albertsen, "Prostate Cancer Diagnosis and Treatment after the Introduction of Prostate-Specific Antigen Screening: 1986–2005," *Journal of the National Cancer Institute* 101, no. 19 (October 2009): 1325–9, http://10.1093/jnci/djp278; H. Gilbert Welch, Steven Woloshin, and Lisa M. Schwartz, "Skin Biopsy Rates and Incidence of Melanoma: Population Based Ecological Study," *BMJ* 331 (2005), http:// https:// doi.org/10.1136/bmj.38516.649537.E0.

6. H. Gilbert Welch et al., "Overstating the Evidence for Lung Cancer Screening: The International Early Lung Cancer Action Program (I-ELCAP) Study," *Archives of Internal*

Medicine 167, no. 21 (2007): 2289–95, http://10.1001 /archinte.167.21.2289.

7. Per-Henrik Zahl, Jan Maehln, and H. Gilbert Welch, "The Natural History of Invasive Breast Cancers Detected by Screening Mammography," *Archives of Internal Medicine* 168, no. 21 (2008): 2311–16, http://doi.org/10.1001 /archinte.168.21.2311.

INDEX

Note: Page numbers in *italics* refer to tables.

Foxglove, 66
Fruits, 140
Fungi, 95. *See also* plant and
mushroom medicines

Gall bladder, 82, 167
Gastric cancer, *115*
Gel state, 24, 25. *See also* intracellular
gel/water
Genes, 9, 10–11, 26, 32, 51, 97. *See
also* oncogene theory, failure of
Genetics, 10, 12, 13, 22, 51, 95
Gerson, Max, 31, 61–65, 67, 118
Gerson therapy
Cardiac glycosides, 67
Coffee enemas, 150
G-strophanthin, 71
Outcomes, 49
Potential therapies, 60–65
Surgery, 135
GI (gastrointestinal) tract, 114
Glacial runoff, 107, 108, 109, 144
Gleevec, 16–17
Glioblastoma, *115*
Gluconeogenesis, 98
Glucose, 19–20, 21, 96, 97–98
Glycolysis, 20, 22, 95–96
Glycolytic pathway, 20, 95
Glyphosate (Roundup), 27, 32, 84,
138
Goethe, Johann Wolfgang von, 27
Goetheanistic observation, 28–30
Goldenseal, 82
Grains, 140
Gravity, 43
Greater celandine, 82
Grounding, 126, 148
Grounding mats, 164
G-strophanthin, 66, 67, 68, 69, 71
Gut flora, 84

Health, working definition of, 27
Heart attack, 69–70
Heart disease, 3, 66, 69–70, 142

Heart failure, 66
Heart of Centering Prayer, 128–129
Heart of Centering Prayer, The
(Bourgeault), 128
Heart-centered choices, 129
Heavy water, 106
Helixor (company), 144–146, 165
Heme molecule, 168
Herbal medicines, 83–84
Homeopathy, 119, 127, 133–134
Hormones, 2–3, 27, 69, 142
Houston, Robert J., 122
Human consciousness, 37, 38, 39,
127–128, 141–142
Human Genome Project, 26
Human Heart, Cosmic Heart
(company), 163, 164, 165, 166
Human Heart, Cosmic Heart
(Cowan), 57, 128
Hydrogen
Deuterium, 105–106, 108, 111
Deuterium-depleted water
(DDW), 110
NADH, 114, 118
Role of, 113
Hyperlipidemia, 58
Hypertension, 58, 142
Hyperthermia, 91
Hyphal form, 120

Immune dysfunction, 58
Immune system, 98, 142, 145
Infections, 58, 82, 83, 91, 142
Infectious disease, 120
Inflammation, 81, 138
Influenza, 3, 58
Inotropic effect, 66
Intracellular gel/water
Deuterium (isotope) and, 107, 109
Distortion of, 64
Electromagnetic fields (EMF), 127
EMF exposure, 146–147
Function of, 25–27
Gelatin, 96–97

INDEX

ABOUT THE AUTHOR

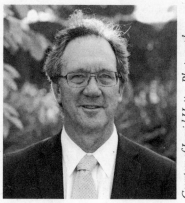

Courtesy of Ingrid Hatton Photography

Thomas Cowan, MD, has studied and written about many subjects in medicine, including nutrition, homeopathy, anthroposophical medicine, and herbal medicine. He is the author of *Vaccines, Autoimmunity, and the Changing Nature of Childhood Illness* and *Human Heart, Cosmic Heart*; principal author of *The Fourfold Path to Healing*; and coauthor (with Sally Fallon) of *The Nourishing Traditions Book of Baby and Child Care*. Dr. Cowan has served as vice president of the Physicians' Association for Anthroposophic Medicine and is a founding board member of the Weston A. Price Foundation. He also writes the "Ask the Doctor" column in *Wise Traditions in Food, Farming, and the Healing Arts* (the Weston A. Price Foundation's quarterly magazine), has lectured throughout the United States and Canada, and is the cofounder of two family businesses, Dr. Cowan's Garden (www.drcowansgarden.com) and Human Heart, Cosmic Heart (www.humanheartcosmicheart.com). He has three grown children and currently practices medicine in San Francisco, where he resides with his wife, Lynda Smith.